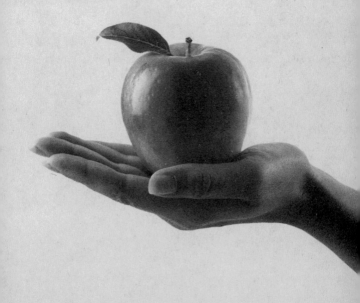

FOCUS ON THE **FAMILY** RESOURCES

7 STEPS TO HEALTHY EATING

PAUL C. REISSER, M.D.

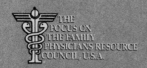

THE FOCUS ON THE FAMILY PHYSICIANS RESOURCE COUNCIL, U.S.A.

Tyndale House Publishers, Inc.
Carol Stream, Illinois

Visit Tyndale's exciting Web site at www.tyndale.com

TYNDALE is a registered trademark of Tyndale House Publishers, Inc.

Tyndale's quill logo is a trademark of Tyndale House Publishers, Inc.

Living Books is a registered trademark of Tyndale House Publishers, Inc.

Focus on the Family is a registered trademark of Focus on the Family, Colorado Springs, Colorado.

7 Steps to Healthy Eating

Designed by Luke Daab

Adapted from the *Complete Guide to Family Health, Nutrition, and Fitness*, ISBN-10: 0-8423-6181-2; ISBN-13: 978-0-8423-6181-1. Copyright © 2006 by Tyndale House Publishers, Inc.

ISBN-13: 978-1-4143-1047-3
ISBN-10: 1-4143-1047-1

Printed in the United States of America

12   11   10   09   08   07   06
7   6   5   4   3   2   1

TABLE OF CONTENTS

Foreword by Dr. James Dobson vii
Acknowledgments xiii

Introduction
Some Food for Thought on Food xvii

1
Go Easy on the Added Sugars 1

2
Gravitate toward Whole Grains 13

3
Consume Fiber Regularly 21

4
Eat Plenty of Fruits and Vegetables 27

5
Get Enough "Good" Fats—and Avoid
the "Bad" 35

6

Choose Supplements Carefully 53

7

Track Your Eating Patterns 67

Afterword
The Importance of
Breaking Bread Together 89

Endnotes 91
Index 93

FOREWORD BY
DR. JAMES DOBSON

August 15, 1990, began much like any other day for me. I awoke early in the morning and headed to the gym for a game of basketball with a group of friends and colleagues—some of whom were as much as twenty or thirty years younger than I! Because I frequently hit the court with these "youngsters," and because I had reached middle age with the lanky build that allowed me to still move easily, I assumed that I was in the prime of physical health.

A sharp pain in my chest on that late summer morning told me otherwise. I excused myself from the game and drove alone to the hospital (something I do *not* recommend to anyone who suspects he or she is experiencing a serious medical problem!). Hoping and praying that I was merely battling fatigue, I knew deep down that there was something else terribly wrong. It didn't take the doctors long to confirm that, sure enough, this "healthy" basketball enthusiast had transformed, in the blink of an eye, into a heart attack victim.

As I lay in the hospital in the days following that ordeal, I realized that, early-morning basketball games notwithstanding, my predicament was directly related to my lifestyle choices and, in particular, the fatty foods I was allowing in my diet. I asked the Lord to give me another chance, resolving to use every resource at my disposal to safeguard my heart and my health through a combination of healthy diet and exercise. Despite some setbacks (I suffered a stroke in 1998 but recovered from it almost immediately), I have endeavored to keep that commitment, and, today, I am feeling better than ever.

Like so many Americans, prior to my heart attack, I was extremely busy—but not necessarily *active* in a way that would ensure optimal physical health. Indeed, statistics show that, despite our frantic pace of living and continued advances in the medical field, Americans suffer from an alarming number of health problems, many of which could be prevented or at least decreased by changing bad habits.

Research confirms just how serious the situation has become. The latest figures from the American Heart Association show that 13 million Americans have coronary heart disease; 5.4 million have suffered a stroke; and 65 million have been diagnosed with high blood pressure. Unfortunately, a large number of these cases are related, at least in part, to lifestyle choices. The AHA also reports that 48.5 million American adults (nearly 23 percent) are smokers. From 1995 to 1999, an average of 442,398 Americans died annually of smoking-related illnesses (32.2 percent of these deaths were cardiovascular related). The American Cancer

Society estimates that 180,000 of the cancer deaths in 2004 could be attributed to smoking. Further, one-third of cancer deaths in 2004 were related to nutrition, physical inactivity, being overweight or obese, and other lifestyle issues. In other words, many of them were *preventable*!

As I suggested earlier, perhaps the biggest factors in maintaining proper physical health are diet and exercise. Unfortunately, a recent study revealed that a full 25 percent of Americans reported participating in *no* physical activity during their leisure time. Perhaps that is why more than 65 percent of adults in the United States are overweight, including 30 percent who are clinically obese. Between 1971 and 2000, the average daily caloric intake for men grew by about 7 percent, which translates into seventeen pounds of additional body fat per year. Obesity dramatically affects life span, as well. The life expectancy of a twenty-year-old white male who is clinically obese decreases by an estimated thirteen years, and for black males, an astonishing average of twenty years are lost due to obesity. One recent study revealed that the number of annual deaths attributable to obesity among adults in the United States is about 300,000. And perhaps most telling of all, airlines are telling us that they now have to carry additional fuel in order to transport more overweight customers.

This situation is sobering, but I am living proof that a dramatic change in eating habits, combined with a focused regimen of heart-strengthening exercise, can significantly improve one's overall health. I'll admit that the prospect of making such radical lifestyle changes can be daunting, but let me assure you that it is worth the investment. Choosing a healthy lifestyle *now*, while you still can, is infinitely preferable to being sidelined by a stroke, heart attack, cancer, or some other health crisis in the future.

This pocket guide and its parent book, the *Complete Guide to Family Health, Nutrition, and Fitness,* are excellent resources designed to answer many of the questions that may arise as you endeavor to put yourself and your loved ones on the road to a healthier life. You'll find information on preventing the three most common health problems—cardiovascular disease, cancer, and diabetes—as well as practical advice on those critical disciplines that I have mentioned several times already: *diet and exercise*. These books can help you discover answers to specific health-related questions for family members of all ages; foster *emotional* and *spiritual* health in addition to physical fitness; and so much more. The information presented here is based on the most up-to-date medical research as well as the firsthand experiences of members of Focus on the Family's Physicians Resource Council.

Perhaps you consider yourself generally healthy and are simply looking for a plan to help you stay that way. Or maybe you or someone you love is dangerously overweight or suffering from a serious health problem related to poor lifestyle choices in the past. Either way, this book will provide you with the tools you need—as a complement to the advice of your personal physician, of course—to live smarter and healthier. Change is never easy, but it is possible, and I pray that God will bless you as you endeavor to be a good steward of the body He has given you.

James C. Dobson

James C. Dobson, Ph.D.

ACKNOWLEDGMENTS

The following members of the Focus on the Family Physicians Resource Council served as primary reviewers for all or parts of this manuscript, and their input, suggestions, and insights have been of critical importance:

BYRON CALHOUN, M.D., F.A.C.O.G., F.A.C.S.
Maternal-Fetal Medicine—Rockford, Illinois

DOUGLAS O. W. EATON, M.D.
Internal Medicine—Loma Linda, California

ELAINE ENG, M.D., F.A.P.A.
Psychiatry—Flushing, New York

J. THOMAS FITCH, M.D., F.A.A.P.
Pediatrics—San Antonio, Texas

DONALD GRABER, M.D.
Psychiatry—Elkhart, Indiana

W. DAVID HAGER, M.D., F.A.C.O.G.
Gynecology—Lexington, Kentucky

DANIEL R. HINTHORN, M.D., F.A.C.P.
Infectious Disease—Kansas City, Kansas

GERARD R. HOUGH, M.D., F.A.A.P.
Pediatrics—Brandon, Florida

GAYLEN M. KELTON, M.D., F.A.A.F.P.
Family Medicine—Indianapolis, Indiana

JOHN P. LIVONI, M.D.
Radiology—Little Rock, Arkansas

ROBERT W. MANN, M.D., F.A.A.P.
Pediatrics—Mansfield, Texas

MARILYN A. MAXWELL, M.D., F.A.A.P.
Internal Medicine/Pediatrics—St. Louis, Missouri

PAUL MEIER, M.D.
Psychiatry—Richardson, Texas

GARY MORSCH, M.D., F.A.A.F.P.
Family Medicine—Olathe, Kansas

MARY ANNE NELSON, M.D.
Family Medicine—Cedar Rapids, Iowa

GREGORY RUTECKI, M.D.
Internal Medicine—Columbus, Ohio

ROY C. STRINGFELLOW, M.D., F.A.C.O.G.
Gynecology—Colorado Springs, Colorado

MARGARET COTTLE, M.D.
Palliative Care—Vancouver, British Columbia

PETER NIEMAN, M.D., F.A.A.P.
Pediatrics—Calgary, Alberta

TYNDALE PUBLISHER

DOUGLAS R. KNOX

EDITORIAL STAFF

PAUL C. REISSER, M.D.
Primary Author

DAVID DAVIS
Managing Editor/Contributing Author

LISA JACKSON
Tyndale Editor

FOCUS ON THE FAMILY

BRADLEY G. BECK, M.D.
Medical Issues Advisor/Research Editor/Contributing Author

VICKI DIHLE, PA-C
Medical Research Analyst/Contributing Author

BARBARA SIEBERT
Manager, Medical Outreach

LINDA BECK
Administrative Support

REGINALD FINGER, M.D.
Medical Issues Analyst

KARA ANGELBECK
Health and Wellness Coordinator

TOM NEVEN
Book Editor

SOME FOOD FOR THOUGHT ON FOOD

Have you ever asked yourself any of the following questions?

For years I've been hearing that fats are bad, and that I should gravitate toward foods that say "low fat" or "nonfat" on the label. Now I'm hearing that carbohydrates are bad and that I should avoid eating them. What gives?

Do I get enough vitamins and minerals from my food, or should I take a supplement?

Every weekend on my local radio station, I hear infomercials for nutritional products that sound too good to be true. Are they?

Sure, I'd like my family to eat healthier foods, but what exactly does that mean, and how do we break some of our bad habits?

It seems like every other month someone comes out with a new surefire way to lose weight. I've tried most of them, and nothing seems to work for long. What am I doing wrong?

I feel tired and irritable most of the time. Should I change something in my diet?

Because we live in a nation blessed with a richer bounty and variety of foods than at any other time or place in history, one would think that deciding what to eat would be a straightforward task. But too many of us don't feel well, or aren't as healthy as we would like, or are overweight. At the same time, we are bombarded every day with advice (half of which seems to contradict the other half) about what we should or shouldn't eat, drink, and take as supplements, accompanied by promises of boundless energy and the Body Beautiful if we will only follow that advice. No wonder we have so many questions!

This book will not set forth imaginative nutritional theories, lists of miracle supplements for you to buy, magic formulas for choosing what you eat, or recommendations that you orient your diet around exotic foods that you may have a hard time swallowing (let alone finding). It will, however, attempt to give you a straightforward, reality-based orientation to the subject of healthy eating, and a handle on some words and catchphrases that you've probably heard but may not understand the significance of. (*What exactly are saturated fats? Why should I avoid trans-fats?*) Hopefully this will help you make better-informed decisions about the foods you buy and prepare for yourself and your family.

You'll be happy to know that steering your family toward healthier eating habits doesn't require that you adopt the motto, "If it tastes good, spit it out!" Furthermore, if you're well aware that the foods you've been choosing aren't exactly the best body fuel—or even if you're a certified junk food addict—you should understand that the seven steps set forth in this book are meant to be just that: seven steps, not a hundred flying leaps. By making gradual adjustments rather than radical changes to your family's diet, your healthy *choices* are more likely to be healthy *habits* that will last for a lifetime. (And, you'll avoid the uproar that is likely to occur if you insist that your family members immediately give up all of their favorite foods.)

A note of explanation before we begin: In this book you'll find a number of references to dietary recommendations published by the Institute of Medicine (or IOM). The IOM is one of four components of the National Academies, a private, nonprofit, nongovernment organization whose mission is to provide reliable health information to citizens, professionals, corporations, and the government. The IOM's reports and recommendations are built upon the best available research and on expert opinion, and they represent an important source of nutritional advice in the United States.

Now, let's take some steps toward healthy eating.

1

GO EASY ON THE
ADDED SUGARS

Contrary to the opinions found in a number of popular
books over the past few decades, sugars aren't the
cause of all disease, the root of all evil, or an imminent
threat to world peace. But they are definitely a poor
quality of fuel for our body, and the dramatic increase
in their consumption in the United States and other
developed countries has been a major step in the
wrong direction. To put it bluntly, most of us could
stand to cut back, and some of us need a major overhaul of our taste buds.

ABOUT SUGAR

Carbohydrates—important nutrients that serve primar-
ily as sources of energy in the body—fall into two basic
categories: simple (commonly called sugars) and complex. Three very important sugars are glucose, fructose,
and sucrose.

- Glucose (also called blood sugar) is the most important
  simple carbohydrate, because it is the primary energy
  source for almost every cell in the body. Our biochemical

machinery is programmed to break down more complex carbohydrates into glucose or to convert the other simple sugars into it.

- Fructose (also called fruit sugar) is the sweetest of the sugars. It is abundant in fruits and honey and is readily converted to glucose.
- Sucrose, which consists of one glucose and one fructose molecule joined together, is the compound that we're usually talking about when we mention dietary sugar.

The complex carbohydrates include important structures that store energy in plants and animals. Starch, which we will discuss in the next chapter, is the general term for a long chain of hundreds or even thousands of glucose molecules linked together and packed into certain parts of plants.

Sugars occur naturally in many foods, but they are also added to many products to enhance sweetness—often with less than desirable results.

Where to find sugar on an ingredient label
Many foods we buy include significant amounts of one or more types of added sugars under a variety of aliases. You might notice some of the following listed among the ingredients of the foods on your shelves.

- Sucrose is also known as white sugar, table sugar, refined sugar, granulated sugar, cane sugar, and beet sugar. A teaspoon of sugar contains about sixteen calories.
- Powdered sugar, also known as confectioners' sugar, is basically white sugar pulverized to a fine consistency, with a little cornstarch added to prevent lumps from forming.

- Raw sugar, or partially refined sugar, is brown and coarser than white sugar. True raw sugar is banned in the United States because it may contain unsavory ingredients such as bacteria and insect parts, but the products sold here (such as Sugar In The Raw or turbinado) have had impurities removed.
- Molasses is the thick, brown syrup produced during the extraction and refining of sugar from cane.
- Brown sugar is white sugar to which molasses has been added.
- Dextrose is another name for glucose.
- Levulose is another name for fructose.
- Invert sugar, a mix of glucose and fructose, occurs naturally (as in honey) or by chemical action on cane sugar.
- Corn syrup is a liquid derived from cornstarch.
- High-fructose corn syrup, a form of corn syrup that was introduced in the mid-1960s, is sweeter than corn syrup, cheaper than sugar obtained from sugar cane (but equally sweet), and not prone to crystallize, making it a popular sweetener that has been added to an enormous number of products. Between 1966 and 2001, high-fructose corn syrup consumption in the United States rose from zero to over sixty pounds per person annually.[1]
- Most forms of honey are sweeter than white sugar. About 220 million pounds (including more than three hundred unique flavors) of honey are produced every year in the United States by more than 2.5 million colonies of honeybees. Each pound of honey represents about 2 million visits to flowers by bees and about fifty thousand flight miles. A tablespoon of honey contains about sixty-four calories (compared to about forty-eight calories in a tablespoon of sugar).

THE TROUBLE WITH SUGAR

A widely quoted report released in 2000 by the United States Department of Agriculture (USDA) raised national eyebrows when it reported that annual sugar consumption in America had reached 158 pounds per person—a whopping fifty teaspoons per day—in 1999, up 30 percent from 1983.

Actually these numbers were based on the amount of sugar available in the wholesale market. Estimates based on surveys of people's eating habits (also conducted by the USDA) revealed somewhat lower (but still impressive) numbers: 109 pounds per year for a typical teenage boy and 64 pounds for the average American citizen.[2]

Why so much? Obviously, we all like one or more sweet foods, and for some of us many of them seem to be addicting. In addition, many foods that are not particularly sweet, such as ketchup, contain a surprising amount of sugar in one of the many forms listed above.

If all the various forms of sugar are so pleasing to the taste buds, how might they cause us trouble? Several noteworthy concerns have been raised about our love affair with sugar.

Sugar and obesity

The number of Americans, young and old, who are overweight or obese has increased dramatically over the past two decades, as has our national consumption of added sugars. Currently Americans on average consume 16 percent of their calories from added sugars. Among children ages six to eleven, the number is 18 percent, while teenagers derive 20 percent of their calories from added sugars. Among the young, soft drinks—what some critics call liquid candy—are a major source of these calories. A typical twelve-ounce canned soft drink contains the equivalent of about ten teaspoons of sugar, yielding 140 calories. This by itself represents the maximum daily intake of added sugars recommended by the USDA. But fast-food restaurants, convenience stores, and movie theaters sell soft drinks in colossal serving sizes ranging from thirty-two to fifty-two ounces, often with free refills. A forty-two-ounce fast-food "supersize" nondiet soft drink packs more than four hundred calories.

The contribution of sweets to obesity may involve more than calorie counts. In many people the metabolic response to surges of blood glucose from products containing a lot of simple sugars appears to promote fat storage. Unfortunately, the same may be happening with many starches and other mainstays of the low-fat approach to eating that has been encouraged by government and health professionals for the past three decades. We will look at this in more detail in the next chapter.

Empty calories
One of the strongest arguments against the wholesale consumption of sugar is that it is basically a raw energy

source without any additional nutritive value. No vitamins, minerals, fiber, or other useful compounds are present in a typical can of soda. Enjoy a medium-sized orange and you get a total of eighty calories, of which about fifty-six come from sugars. But the orange also contains 7 grams of fiber, a gram of protein, a generous dose of vitamin C, and some vitamin A, iron, and calcium. Polish off a mere five ounces of a typical orange soda—less than half of a twelve-ounce can—and you get the same number of calories, all from sugar in one form or another, plus a little caffeine to jangle your nerves and—that's all, folks! Drink the entire can, and you'll consume twice as many calories as the orange contains. Of course, using artificial sweeteners is one way to indulge your sweet tooth without consuming empty calories, but some have questioned their safety.

Sugar vs. the teeth

Actually, this isn't just a shortcoming of sugar. Carbohydrates in any form serve as a food supply for bacteria within the mouth that produce enamel-eroding acid. What makes a carbohydrate bad for the teeth isn't necessarily how sweet it is—the bacteria can be as happy with raisins as with candy—but how long it hangs around inside the mouth. Sticky, sugary foods are thus likely to be troublemakers, especially for those who don't brush after every meal. In general, the greater the percentage of one's daily calories that comes in the form of sugars, the greater the risk of dental caries (tooth decay).

Sugar and hyperactivity

The popular notion that hyperactivity or aggressive behavior in children is provoked by eating sugar has persisted for decades, despite a lack of any consistent support from scientific research. Numerous studies evaluating behavior and learning among children given variable amounts of sugar and artificial sweeteners have shown minimal, if any, objective impact. If Johnny seems "amped up" after a few rounds of soft drinks, cake, and ice cream at a friend's birthday party, the sugar he gobbled up might seem like a prime suspect. But the general excitement, games, presents, and per- haps the caffeine lurking in the sodas are more likely to blame. Nevertheless, if parents notice that a child's behavior seems to take a turn for the worse whenever sugary foods cross his lips, it certainly wouldn't hurt him to stay away from them.

HOW MUCH IS TOO MUCH?

Current recommendations from the U.S. Department of Agriculture call for limiting the day's amount of added sugars to less than 10 percent of your total daily calo- ries. This translates to a daily intake of 24 grams (the equivalent of six teaspoons of table sugar) for 1,600 calories, 40 grams (ten teaspoons, the amount in one twelve-ounce soft drink) for 2,000 calories, and 56 grams (fourteen teaspoons) for 2,400 calories. Remember that *these amounts don't apply to the sugars that occur naturally in foods such as fruit and milk.*

You can tally the number of grams of sugar in any packaged product at the store by checking the Nutrition Facts label. Unfortunately, this does not distinguish between naturally occurring and added sugars. Often the nature of the product leaves little doubt: In a soft drink, you can be certain that all 40 or so grams of the sugar were added, while in an orange all of the 12 or more grams of sugar were there to start with. On the other hand, a cup of raw blueberries contains 14 grams of natural sugar, while a cup of frozen sweetened blueberries contains 45 grams of sugar. The Nutrition Facts label wouldn't tell you that 31 grams were added.

HOW DO I CONTROL THE SUGAR FLOW?

If your family includes one or more members who are big fans of sweets, declaring a sudden moratorium in the name of good health may lead to a minor revolt. All of the following approaches are helpful, but they may be more successful if phased in over time.

1. On packaged foods, check the ingredient list for added sugar, whether named directly or under one of its many aliases. Try to avoid foods in which some

form of added sugar is the first or second ingredient on the list.

2. Some major sources of sugar (and calories) are those perennial favorites: cakes, pies, cookies, pastries, and candies. They won't kill anyone if eaten once in a while, but daily dosing should be avoided. Fruit is a better option for dessert.

3. Watch the sugar content of breakfast cereals, and choose brands that contain less than 8 grams per serving. (The Nutrition Facts label comes in handy here. See chapter 7 for more on how to read the Nutrition Facts.)

4. You have a much easier time shaping the taste preferences of a baby who is just beginning to explore the world of foods beyond milk, compared with a ten-year-old who is already a confirmed lover of candy and soft drinks. Steer the growing toddler and preschooler toward fruit as a dessert, rather than cake and ice cream, and toward unsweetened cereal rather than Chocolate Frosted Sugar Wads.

5. A soft drink may be hard to resist at a ball game or the movies, but otherwise you should limit the number of soft drinks you—and especially your kids—consume every week. Of particular concern among children and teenagers is the replacement of other nutrients with the empty calories in soft drinks. Among teenagers, carbonated soft drinks supply 9 percent of daily calories among boys and 8 percent

in girls' diets. One study of the eating habits of children found that those who drank the most soft drinks also ate the least amount of fruits and vegetables. For children, milk is a better option (unless they are lactose intolerant).

6. While various fruit-flavored beverages may seem like a healthier alternative to soft drinks, most of these contain a small percentage of actual fruit juice (if any) and a lot of sugar. (Think soft drinks without the fizz.) If you're not sure, check the label for the amount of juice—and the amount of sugar.

7. Surprisingly, even pure fruit juice usually provides little more than the sugars found in the fruit, some vitamin C, and perhaps a little calcium if it's fortified. In babies and young children, fruit juice is not an appropriate substitute for breast milk, formula, or (after the first birthday) cow's milk. Those who come to favor juice over better sources of nutrition can develop diarrhea and gas, and may become malnourished. The following guidelines will allow children to enjoy fruit juice without becoming "juicaholics" or damaging their teeth:

• Infants younger than six months of age should not be given fruit juices at all. Indeed, you would be wise to avoid feeding juice to any infant or toddler from a bottle; wait until he can take it from a cup.

• Limit juice intake to four to six ounces per day for children six and younger. Starting at age seven, you can set the limit at eight to twelve ounces per day. If he wants more than the daily limit, dilute juice with an equal amount of water.

- Don't allow an infant or child to go to sleep sucking on a bottle containing juice, milk, or any other liquid that contains sugar. This not only promotes tooth decay but can also increase the risk for developing an ear infection.
- Encourage children to eat whole fruit, which contains fewer calories and more fiber per serving than juice.
- Since citrus fruits may provoke allergic responses during the first year, consider withholding orange juice until after the first birthday. (Check with your baby's doctor.)

2

GRAVITATE TOWARD WHOLE GRAINS

Grains are the small, dry, one-seed fruit of cereal grasses—wheat, rice, corn, oats, and barley. We think of cereal, of course, as what we pour out of a box for breakfast, but a wondrous variety of foods derived from cereal grasses have fed the human race for millennia. Grains contain starches (an important form of complex carbohydrate). Before we discuss the importance of whole-grain foods—as opposed to those that are refined or processed—it's important to understand a bit about starches and the benefits of including them in our diet (or the ills of including too much of them).

STARCHES: "THEY FATTEN ME, THEY FATTEN ME NOT"

Starches are packed into certain parts of a variety of foods, including grains, legumes (the bean and pea family, plus lentils and peanuts), and tubers (root vegetables such as potatoes and yams). These foods have been the staple of cultivation around the world because they are both generous and generally inexpensive sources of carbohydrate fuel that can be prepared and consumed in a variety of ways. Their lack of fat content has given them a particularly esteemed status in the United States over the past thirty years, as dietary recommendations from government and professional groups stressed the importance of eating low-fat or nonfat foods.

In the early 1990s, starch-containing foods such as bread, cereal, rice, and pasta were given a prominent position at the base of the Food Guide Pyramid, a diagram created by the U.S. Department of Agriculture and the U.S. Department of Health and Human Services to illustrate which foods should (and shouldn't) be the cornerstone of our diet. The original pyramid recommended six to eleven servings of starch-containing foods every day, while the revised (2005) Food Guide Pyramid suggests five to eight "ounce equivalents" of the grain group for adults. (See pages 74–77 and http://www.mypramid.gov.) So why would a host of weight-loss programs such as the Atkins diet, Sugar Busters! and Protein power arrive at the conculsion that these foods are responsibile for a host of dietary ills?

To address that question, we need to take a closer look at what happens when we consume these foods. Traditionally, complex carbohydrate foods (including all of the various forms of starches) have been considered timed-release sources of fuel. Eat a candy bar or drink a soda, and one can reasonably assume that the sugars it contains will gain rapid access to the bloodstream. (Indeed, they usually do.) Have a piece of bread or a baked potato, on the other hand, and it will take a while to disassemble all of those complex molecules and release their glucose into circulation—or will it? Depending upon what happened between their harvest and their arrival at the table, the constituents of many complex carbohydrate foods may be capable of releasing large amounts of glucose into the bloodstream very rapidly—even more rapidly, in fact, than sugar itself.

A measurement called the glycemic index (or GI) has been utilized in recent years (though more widely among dietary professionals in Canada, Europe, and Australia than in the United States) as an estimate of the tendency of a food to raise blood glucose. Glucose, the reference food, is given a GI of 100. For other foods, a GI of 70 or more is considered high; one less than 55 is considered low; and one between 55 and 70 is intermediate.

What kinds of carbohydrate foods have the highest glycemic index? One would expect candy and soft drinks to lead the pack. They are indeed on the higher end of the list (especially jelly beans). But all of the following foods have a higher GI than white sugar: white, whole wheat, and rye bread; bagels; waffles; mashed, baked, or french fried potatoes; cornflakes; instant rice; corn chips and pretzels. What foods tend to have a lower glycemic index? With few exceptions, vegetables, fruits (except dried dates), and legumes (peas and beans); pumpernickel and heavy, mixed-grain breads; milk and low-fat yogurt; and (surprise) most pastas, especially when lightly cooked (the so-called al dente style).

What is it about certain foods that raises their glycemic index? Obviously, an abundance of simple sugars has an impact. But the preparation of many starch-laden foods (for example, baking or mashing potatoes) alters their physical characteristics in a way that allows them to be converted into glucose very rapidly. Unfortunately, one of the most common alterations of food over the past century—the processing and refining of grains, especially wheat and rice—significantly raises the GI of these everyday staples. For example, the outer bran and inner germ layers are removed from wheat in order to increase efficiency and stability in creating white flour, which may in turn be finely ground. These characteristics all lead to more rapid digestion and conversion into glucose, and thus more dramatic changes in blood sugar after these foods are eaten.

Many factors impact how rapidly blood glucose changes after a meal. These include:

- **How much of a food is eaten.** Carrots have a moderately high glycemic index, but one would have to eat a huge number to provoke a dramatic effect on blood glucose.
- **What else is eaten with the food.** We rarely eat just one food at a time for a meal. If a high–glycemic index

carbohydrate is eaten with some protein and fat, absorption of the entire mix tends to be slower.

- **Individual characteristics** of the eater (such as age) may alter the rate at which food is digested and absorbed.
- **The presence of fiber.** Foods that are rich in fiber, such as vegetables and most fruits, are the true timed-release sources of fuel. (Note that riper fruits tend to have a higher sugar content and thus a higher glycemic index.) Whole-grain breads, which are more abundant in fiber than their refined counterparts, may have a similar glycemic index if the flour has been finely ground. However, the benefits of their nutrients and fiber counterbalance the impact of their glycemic index.

If a food has a high glycemic index, does that make it bad? While some advocates of low-carbohydrate diets seem to imply that high-glycemic foods are literal poison, the picture isn't quite that black-and-white. Carrots, beets, bananas, cantaloupe, papayas, and pineapples, for example, have a moderately high GI, but that hardly qualifies them as foods to be avoided at all cost. Indeed, another factor that must be considered along with the glycemic index is the *amount* of carbohydrate in a given serving of food. The *glycemic load* is obtained by dividing the glycemic index of a food by 100 and then multiplying it by the number of grams of carbohydrate in that portion. Dietitians note that the glycemic load is equally if not more important than the glycemic index. For example, even though a medium-sized carrot has a relatively high glycemic index of 92, it contains only about 4 grams of carbohydrate, so its glycemic load is 3.7. Mashed potato has a similar glycemic index of 97, but a typical serving contains about 23 grams of carbohydrate, for which the glycemic load is 22—six times greater than that of the carrot.

That being said, a diet heavy on high-glycemic foods—especially those that are calorie dense and have little additional nutritional value—could cause problems for many people because of the physiological response that they are likely to provoke. Eating foods that provoke a rapid rise in blood glucose causes the pancreas to release a surge of insulin so that the glucose can be escorted into all of the cells that need it. But there are some downsides to this response: First, a relatively rapid rise and fall of glucose may provoke hunger, which leads to—that's right—more eating. In fact, the hunger may last well after the blood glucose has risen again. If the desire for more food leads to another round of high–glycemic index treats, the cycle may repeat itself. Second, insulin not only moves glucose into cells. It also promotes storage of any excess calories as fat and slows the use of fat as a source of energy.

THE GOODNESS OF WHOLE GRAINS

The tendency for foods derived from processed and refined grain products to affect blood sugar in unfavorable ways isn't the only reason why whole grains are better for you than those that have been refined (an ironic term for this process):

Fiber, vitamins, and minerals are lost during refining and processing (though some are replaced). Whole-grain products contain a variety of useful compounds, including phytochemicals (see pages 31 and 33), anti-oxidants, folic acid, B vitamins, iron, and vitamin E. (See chapter 6 for more on the role of vitamins.)

A number of studies have shown a link between eating whole grains and a lower risk of developing cardio-vascular disease, diabetes, and cancer.[3]

In addition, whole-grain foods generally have a more generous supply of dietary fiber. (We will discuss the many benefits of dietary fiber in the next chapter.)

HOW CAN I GET MORE WHOLE GRAINS INTO MY DAILY FOOD ROUTINE?

1. Buy whole-grain bread or other baked products, including crackers. Check the ingredient list for whole wheat, whole oats, whole rye, whole barley, whole cornmeal, etc., or a combination of these in a multigrain product. The term *cracked wheat* also is a good sign, referring to whole wheat grains that have been cut or crushed, and *graham flour* refers to flour made from the entire wheat grain (also called the wheat berry). The term *wheat flour*, on the other hand, doesn't tell you whether it's whole wheat or a refined version. (Keep in mind that the presence of

whole-grain ingredients isn't the only item on your mental checklist. A whole-grain cracker, for example, may also contain trans fats that would be good to avoid.)

2. Similarly, buy cereals made from whole grains. As with baked products, check the ingredient list and look for one or more of the whole grains as the first ingredient. Note that oatmeal is a whole grain, but *old-fashioned* or *steel-cut* oats are less processed than instant versions.

3. Eat brown rather than white rice.

4. When baking, try substituting whole wheat flour for a quarter to a half of the flour needed in the recipe.

5. Look for pasta made from whole wheat or from half whole and half refined wheat.

3

CONSUME FIBER REGULARLY

Dietary fiber, the other major type of complex carbohydrate, plays a supportive but very important role in nutritional health. Fiber is the component of plant foods that we cannot digest. Soluble fiber partially dissolves in water, while insoluble fiber does not. Sources of soluble fiber include many fruits (apples, pears, and strawberries), legumes (peas, beans, and lentils), oatmeal, and oat bran. Sources of insoluble fiber include many vegetables (carrots, celery, tomatoes, zucchini), whole-grain breads and cereals (especially whole wheat), wheat bran, brown rice, and couscous. Soluble or not, since we can't use fiber for energy or building materials, what good is it?

WHAT DOES FIBER DO FOR OUR BODY?

Fiber contributes to the time release of energy from carbohydrates by slowing both the release of food from the stomach and the absorption of digestible carbohydrate that accompanies it. This tends to prevent the spikes in blood glucose and insulin that are undesirable features of high–glycemic index foods (see chapter 2). Foods with a healthy component of fiber tend to have a lower glycemic index. A diet high in fiber may reduce the risk of developing type 2 diabetes.

Fiber can help reduce overeating and weight gain. Slowing the speed with which you consume a meal is a basic strategy in controlling the size of your food portions, and meals higher in fiber content generally take longer to eat. Their larger bulk, increased even more by water they absorb, creates a feeling of fullness. Furthermore, they slow not only the stomach's rate of emptying food but also the passage of food through the small intestine, thus prolonging the sense of being full or even "stuffed."

Fiber (especially the insoluble form) tends to soften and increase the bulk of stool and helps to move it through the colon more rapidly. It thus can prevent or relieve constipation, the most common intestinal complaint in the United States (especially among the elderly). Wheat and oat bran appear to be particularly effective at this, as is psyllium seed, derived from a Mediterranean plant, which swells and becomes gelatinous when moist. Psyllium seed is used in many bulk laxatives such as Metamucil.

Fiber (again, especially the insoluble type) helps prevent diverticulosis, a common condition in which small pouches called diverticula form in the wall of the colon. Diverticula can bleed, become infected (a condition called diverticulitis), or even perforate, resulting in a serious infection within the abdomen. The soft, bulky stools produced by fiber in the diet are also less likely to form small, hard pellets that can lodge in the opening of the appendix, the first step in the development of appendicitis.

Some studies have shown lower rates of colon cancer in populations that consume large amounts of fiber, compared with those on a low-fiber diet. A reasonable explanation for this is that any potential carcinogenic (cancer-inducing) agents arriving in the intestine would be diluted and swept along by soft, bulky stools, and thus not allowed to have prolonged contact with the cells lining the colon. However, other research (including a Harvard study that followed eighty thousand women over sixteen years[4]) has not supported this particular benefit from eating dietary fiber.

Finally, dietary fiber—especially soluble fiber found in oats (including oatmeal and oat bran) and apples—can lower blood cholesterol to a modest degree. This occurs when cholesterol floating through the digestive tract binds to the fiber and is carried out of the body in stool, rather than being absorbed. While the impact of dietary fiber on blood cholesterol levels is usually not as dramatic as may be seen with weight loss or medications, it has been demonstrated to reduce the risk for coronary artery disease.

HOW MUCH FIBER SHOULD I EAT EVERY DAY?

The Institute of Medicine of the National Academies recommends the following daily amounts:

- For adults fifty and younger: 38 grams for men and 25 grams for women.
- For adults fifty-one and older: 30 grams for men and 21 grams for women.[5]

In addition, for children two and older, the current recommendation for fiber intake is an amount in grams equal to their age plus five.

Unfortunately, Americans on average consume about half this amount of fiber or less on a day-to-day basis. If you are interested in tracking your fiber intake, one way to begin is by paying attention to the Nutrition Facts label found on every packaged food. As we will see later in chapter 7, this label includes all sorts of useful tidbits, including grams of fiber per serving. (Of course, you have to note what the label identifies as a serving, and how many servings you are consuming at a given meal.)

HOW CAN I INCREASE MY DAILY DOSE OF FIBER?

The richest sources of dietary fiber are legumes (beans and peas), vegetables and fruits, and whole-grain products. You'll find less of it in refined grain products (white bread and cereals that aren't whole grain), and none in dairy or meat products. Here are a few ways to increase your family's daily dose of fiber:

1. Buy bread that lists whole grain (wheat or otherwise) as the first ingredient on the label, with at least 3 grams of fiber per slice. These tend to be heavier, darker, and more flavorful. If you bake your own bread, use whole-grain flour for a fourth to a half (or more) of the amount of flour in your recipe. (You will need more yeast or baking powder—about a teaspoon more baking powder for every three cups of whole-grain flour.)

2. Look for breakfast cereals with 5 grams or more of fiber per serving. Often they include the words *bran* or *fiber* in the name or display it on the packaging, but check the Nutrition Facts label to see how much fiber is actually present. (Remember also that fiber content may not be the only virtue a cereal offers.) If these cereals don't suit your taste, try adding some unprocessed wheat bran to the cereals you like.

3. Try some whole-grain variations on common products, such as brown rice (rather than white) and whole wheat spaghetti, which contains more than twice the fiber found in regular spaghetti.

4. Add more peas, beans, and lentils, which are among the richest sources of dietary fiber, to your daily routine.

5. Last, but certainly not least, eat a lot of fruits (at least three to four servings) and vegetables (four to five

servings) every day. (For children two to six, at least two fruit and three vegetable servings per day.) Good sources of fiber among fruits include berries, pears, prunes, raisins, strawberries, peaches, oranges, apricots, bananas, and apples. Good vegetable sources of fiber include spinach, artichoke, brussels sprouts, carrots, and corn, as well as the tubers: potatoes and sweet potatoes.

If you have access to the Internet, you can look up the fiber content of foods at the U.S. Department of Agriculture's National Nutrient Database Web site at http://www.nal.usda.gov/fnic/foodcomp/search/. The database allows you to view all of the nutritional characteristics of a specific food. And for each nutrient you can get a listing of its content in hundreds of foods, arranged either alphabetically or by the amount of the nutrient, from most to least.

If your eating habits up to this point have not included much fiber, you will want to make changes gradually. A sudden increase in your daily intake may provoke a few unpleasant responses from your intestinal tract, including cramping, bloating, and gas. If you find yourself getting constipated, drink more fluids, since fiber must absorb water to become soft and bulky.

4

EAT PLENTY OF FRUITS AND VEGETABLES

You've heard this from your mother, your health education teacher, the American Dietetic Association, the government, and hopefully your doctor. Fruits and vegetables are supposed to be good for us (and they are), but they're nearly always the side dish rather than the main event at a meal. (How many times have you picked up the menu at a typical restaurant and found a list of fruit and vegetable entrees?) Since 1991, the "5 A Day for Better Health" program, a joint project of several large federal agencies and private organizations, has been promoting the idea that we should eat five to nine servings of fruit and vegetables every day. But according to the Centers for Disease Control and Prevention's Behavior Risk Factor Surveillance System telephone survey (the world's largest telephone survey), as of 2000 fewer than one in four Americans was actually following this advice, and one in three was consuming only one or two servings every day.

WHAT CONSTITUTES A SERVING OF FRUIT OR VEGETABLE?

Many people struggle to eat enough fruits and vegetables each day. The old Food Guide Pyramid recommended five to nine daily servings, which is a good number to try to reach. Although the new Food Pyramid guidelines make recommendations in terms of specific amounts (for example, cups or ounces), many people still think of fruits and vegetables in terms of servings. But what constitutes a serving?

- Six ounces (three-quarters of a cup) of fruit or vegetable juice.
- One medium-sized whole fruit (such as an orange, apple, or banana).
- One-quarter cup of dried fruit.
- One-half cup of raw, frozen, or cooked vegetables or fruit (sliced or chopped).
- One cup of raw leafy vegetables. Note that a large salad may contain three cups of greens and thus count as three servings.

These amounts reflect the most typical portion sizes determined by surveys of food consumption carried out by the USDA. (In other words, these are amounts that people typically eat.) You may find it interesting to get a measuring cup and see how much you actually serve or eat, compared with these amounts. You may notice that a helping of your favorite vegetable looks more like two servings rather than one. This can help you gauge your daily intake in light of these recommendations.

Some foods are easier to measure than others. Foods that you prepare in small pieces will fit into your measuring cup, but large broccoli spears won't. Here's what constitutes a serving for a few odd-sized items:

- Asparagus: six medium spears
- Broccoli: two spears
- Brussels sprouts: four sprouts
- Carrots: one medium-sized or eight baby-sized carrots
- Celery: two medium stalks
- Dates (dried): five dates
- Grapefruit: half of a medium grapefruit
- Strawberries: seven medium berries

Note: For smaller children, portion sizes will of course be smaller. Two- and three-year-olds, for example, will consume about half of the serving size that would be appropriate for adults. Remember to be cautious about excessive fruit-juice consumption in kids. (See pages 10–11.) For that matter, remember that fruit juice, nutritious as it may be, contains more sugar and calories than the fruit itself and little if any fiber.

SOME HEALTH BENEFITS OF EATING FRUITS AND VEGETABLES

Why eat so many fruits and vegetables? Because Mom was right: An impressive and growing body of research supports her opinion that fruits and vegetables are good for you. Specifically, they can help reduce your risk of some common health problems:

Cancer. More than two hundred studies conducted in various corners of the world support a fundamental conclusion: A diet plentiful in fruits and vegetables tends to protect you from at least some forms of cancer. This is not a universal effect. Not every food derived from plants is protective, and those that appear to offer some protection do not do so against every cancer. Nevertheless, reasonable evidence suggests that regular intake of certain fruits and vegetables may reduce the risk for developing cancer of the mouth, throat, esophagus, lung, colon, and prostate.[6]

Heart disease and stroke. A growing body of evidence supports the idea that a diet rich in a variety of fruits and vegetables may protect against these common and devastating conditions. One major study conducted by the Harvard School of Public Health, for example, found that eating five servings of fruits and vegetables per day was associated with a 30 percent reduction in the risk of stroke in healthy men and women.[7] Another Harvard study found that adults who took eight or more servings of fruits and vegetables every day had 20 percent less heart disease compared to those who ate three or fewer servings per day. Furthermore, the study suggested that for each serving added every day, the risk dropped by 4 percent.[8]

Cataract and macular degeneration. A number of studies suggest that regularly eating dark, leafy green vegetables (such as spinach and kale) may reduce the risk of developing these common eye conditions. While cataracts—clouded lenses within the eye—can be removed and replaced with clear ones, there is no effective treatment for most cases of macular degeneration, the leading cause of blindness among those over sixty-five.

Fruits and vegetables don't walk and talk (except in cartoons), but that doesn't mean they are not amazingly complex. Nutritional science has identified a number of substances found in plants that do more than provide basic nutrients (carbohydrate, protein, and fat) for fuel and building materials. Some of these, such as vitamins C and E, are familiar to us. Others, with tongue-twisting names such as carotenoids and isothiocyanates, belong to a diverse group of compounds called phytochemicals. These are not necessary for life or health (as are the vitamins), but many of them appear to have a protective effect against cancer and heart disease. Needless to say, researchers have only scratched the surface of this biological treasure trove. Furthermore, because of complicated interactions between various substances in fruits and vegetables, the most diligent human effort to reproduce or extract some useful "essence" of a plant for a surefire supplement usually doesn't come close to delivering the goods that are readily available by eating the real thing. We will look at vitamins and supplements in more detail in chapter 6.

HOW CAN I EAT MORE FRUITS AND VEGETABLES?

How can we incorporate more of these foods into our diet? Here are some practical suggestions:

1. Add some mixed frozen vegetables to your favorite soup as you heat it.
2. Enhance your salads with some pieces of fruit.
3. While most of us are used to the typical meat/starch/vegetable combination for a meal, try a second vegetable instead of the potato/rice/pasta.
4. If you order a pizza for take-out or delivery to your home, order a salad with it or make one before it arrives. While you're at it, add a fruit or vegetable to balance out the meal.
5. If the prospect of putting a salad together from scratch provokes you to reach for something simpler (like a box of macaroni), think about buying some precut salad mixes at the store. They're not as economical as using the original ingredients—you're paying for the convenience, after all—but they may be worth it if they increase your family's consumption of greens.
6. Encourage your family (and yourself) to munch on carrot and/or celery sticks instead of chips for appetizers or snacks.
7. Keep some fresh fruit in a bowl in the kitchen or family room for a healthy snack.
8. Add slices of fruit to your favorite cereal. Be adventurous with the types that you try.

9. Serve fruit with dessert . . . or as dessert.

10. For a treat on a hot day, think about fixing or buying a fruit smoothie rather than a milk shake.

11. Try to eat a variety of colors every day. The beautiful colors found in fruits and vegetables are not merely decorative touches. It appears that phytochemicals associated with different colors of fruits and vegetables provide a variety of health benefits. If you limit yourself to products bearing only one or two colors, you'll miss out. Here are a few of the benefits associated with each color:

- Green: Green leafy vegetables are a good source of folic acid, which helps reduce injury to the linings of arteries and the formation of blood clots in the wrong places. Another compound found in green vegetables such as spinach, celery, and avocados is lutein, which may be protective against eye disorders, especially cataracts and macular degeneration.

- Yellow/orange: Many fruits and vegetables of this color carry antioxidants that may protect against cancer and other diseases. (We will look at the importance of antioxidants in chapter 6.)

- Red: Tomatoes and all of their various products (juice, soup, and sauce, among others) are technically fruits, but usually grouped with vegetables. They contain an abundant supply of lycopene, a powerful antioxidant that may protect against cancer (especially cancer of the prostate) and preserve the integrity of blood vessels, among many other benefits.

- Blue/purple: Familiar fruits (and less familiar

vegetables) of this color are also known for containing antioxidants.

- White/tan/brown: Perhaps the least colorful of fruits and vegetables, these are no less healthful. For example, certain foods of the garlic and onion family may lower cholesterol levels and reduce the risk of some types of cancer.

GET ENOUGH "GOOD" FATS—AND AVOID THE "BAD"

We have been told for decades that we should eat as little fat as possible and that doing so will keep us thin, but that approach hasn't always worked. And now we hear other voices saying that eating fat is okay, and that doing so with gusto is apparently the way to lose weight. To complicate matters, the fat in so many of our favorite foods gives them the texture and flavor that we enjoy.

As it turns out, we need a certain amount of fat in both our diet and our body to live well. Fat is actually a member of a family of compounds called lipids, although we commonly use the word *fats* to refer to the entire group. The other members are sterols, which include cholesterol and phospholipids. All of these play a variety of important roles, including:

Energy storage. Our bodies are designed to thrive when food is plentiful and survive when it isn't. One ingenious safeguard is the storage of extra calories in a layer of tissue, which literally covers our body beneath the skin and is also found within the abdomen. This tissue consists of unique cells (called adipose or fat cells) that can store almost unlimited amounts of fuel in the form of fat for immediate and future use. While other types of cells (such as liver or muscle cells) can store only a limited amount of fat, adipose cells can dramatically enlarge to accommodate whatever fat is available to them. One unfortunate result is that a human being can accumulate hundreds of pounds of adipose tissue, to his or her peril.

Protection and appearance. The layer of fat that covers our body from one end to the other has several important functions beyond storing calories for the winter. It serves as a shock absorber for any part of the body that strikes, or is struck by, a blunt object. A wad of fat under the kidneys helps cushion those critical organs from injury when we jump or are jarred. Adipose tissue serves as insulation against external heat and cold. And a certain amount of fat is necessary to give our body an appealing shape.

Structural and functional roles. Among other things, different types of lipids make up the boundary of the cell known as the cell membrane, aid the rapid transmission of nerve impulses throughout the body, and contribute to the formation of bones and sex hormones.

SOME BASIC FAT VOCABULARY

You've probably heard that saturated fats and trans fats aren't good for you, and perhaps you're aware that omega-3 fatty acids and fish oils possess some sort of health benefit. If you look at food labels, you may see terms such as *polyunsaturated* and *partially hydrogenated* applied to a variety of products such as vegetable oils. Many of these ninety-nine-cent words have become part of our vocabulary, but how do they affect our health? In this section we'll introduce you to these different types of fats and discuss the effects they have on our body—both good and bad.

Cholesterol

For all the negative press it receives, one might imagine that cholesterol is rat poison under an assumed name. In fact, it is an important and necessary compound—but one for which there can definitely be too much of a good thing. Cholesterol is necessary for the formation and maintenance of the complex membranes that surround every cell in our body. It is also a component of bile, the liquid formed by the liver that helps disperse fat molecules in the intestine so that they can be absorbed.

About 85 percent of the cholesterol in our body—in fact, all that you can possibly use—is generated internally, mostly by the liver, in quantities affected dramatically both by our genetics and our weight. The rest comes from animal sources in our diet: meats (especially liver and kidney), eggs, fish, and dairy products.

Cholesterol is not soluble in water, which has some major implications for our health. Think of what happens when you pour a little vegetable oil into a pan of water: The oil clumps into droplets and dollops of various sizes and floats to the surface. Blood is essentially a water-based liquid. If cholesterol molecules were released directly into the bloodstream, they would likewise form clumps and would not disperse to all of the cells that need them. Instead, cholesterol molecules are escorted through the bloodstream by carrier proteins that *are* water/blood soluble. These proteins along with various combinations of lipid molecules are packaged together to form lipoproteins, which researchers have sorted into categories based on their density. Two of these—the low-density lipoproteins (or LDL) and the high-density lipoproteins (or HDL)—are particularly important to our health.

LDL packages are larger, lighter, and loaded with more cholesterol. They also have an unfortunate tendency to deposit cholesterol in the walls of arteries, contributing to the buildup of blood-blocking plaque. HDL packages, on the other hand, are smaller and heavier, and carry more protein and less cholesterol than LDL. More important, they help "clean up the mess" left by LDL, removing some of the excess cholesterol and other lipids from tissues and bringing them back to the liver. An abundance of research has shown that the more cholesterol you have associated with LDL, the more likely your arteries are to be congested. The more you have riding on HDL, the more you will be protected from this problem. It's not uncommon to hear about "bad" cholesterol, referring to that which is attached to LDL, and "good" cholesterol that rides with HDL. In fact, cholesterol is cholesterol, but what makes it "good" or "bad" depends a lot on how much you have in circulation and the company it keeps.

Saturated fats and trans fatty acids

A certain type of fat will be called saturated or unsaturated based on the type of fatty acid that is most abundant within it. Saturated fats (SFAs) are the form that the body prefers to store for future energy needs, and so not surprisingly they are abundant in animal fat. Solid or waxy at room temperature, they have been generally considered the "bad guys" in the world of fats, although they are present in some of America's favorite foods—red meats, butter, cheese, whole milk, and ice cream—as well as coconut, palm, and other tropical oils. The primary concern about eating a lot of saturated fats, other than their rich supply of calories, is that they increase cholesterol levels—in particular, the LDL or "bad" cholesterol—and are associated with a higher risk of developing congested arteries that can lead to heart attack or stroke. The American Heart

Association and other organizations recommend that 10 percent or less of our daily calories come from saturated fat.

Monounsaturated fatty acids (MUFAs) turn a "bad fat" into a "good fat" (or at least a "better fat"). MUFAs are found in abundance in olive oil, canola oil, and peanut oil, as well as avocados and most nuts. They are liquid at room temperature but may solidify if refrigerated. They can be used by our body as fuel nearly as efficiently as saturated fats (SFAs), but unlike SFAs they appear to *reduce* cholesterol (LDL or "bad" cholesterol in particular), and may even raise HDL ("good") cholesterol—more on this in a moment. MUFAs may also affect clotting in a beneficial way (that is, reduce the tendency to form unwanted blood clots in arteries).

Polyunsaturated fats (PUFAs) are liquid both at room temperature and in the refrigerator and, like monounsaturated fats, tend to lower cholesterol when substituted for saturated fatty acids. Indeed, a few decades ago this selling point led to a widespread shift from butter to various forms of margarine derived from polyunsaturated oils, on the assumption that these would be healthier for the heart. (There is, however, more to that story.) PUFAs also are important components of cell membranes and are used by our body in the synthesis of important hormones. Food sources that are rich in PUFAs include vegetable oils made from corn, safflower, cottonseed, flaxseed, soybean, sunflower, and others, as well as fish oils.

One definite liability of polyunsaturated fats is that they are susceptible to a process called oxidation, a chemical reaction that causes them to deteriorate and become rancid. Exposure to light, air, and heat speeds this process. If you leave butter, olive oil, and your favorite polyunsaturated oil sitting in an open dish, the butter will be the last to go rancid because its fat is saturated, so the oxidation proceeds much more slowly. Olive oil, which contains more monounsaturated fatty acids (MUFAs) will be the second of the three to develop that nasty, rancid aroma. The polyunsaturated oil will be the fastest of the three to go bad, especially if the surroundings are warm. This tendency toward oxidation and rancidity can cause foods full of polyunsaturated fats to become unappetizing. It may also make them hazardous, because the oxidation process makes them potentially dangerous to cells in a variety of ways.

Food manufacturers realized that this particular drawback of polyunsaturated fatty acids could be countered if they could make them less "PUFA-like"—in other words, if they could make these fatty acids behave more like saturated fats. Adding hydrogen atoms to PUFAs in a limited fashion yields fats that are called partially hydrogenated—a term that you will see on many food labels. This not only stabilizes PUFAs so that they won't go rancid, but it also converts liquid oils into more solid, spreadable, and generally more appealing products. Sounds good so far, but unfortunately research now suggests that the law of unintended consequences may be at work, canceling whatever benefits partially hydrogenated polyunsaturated fats might otherwise offer. In fact, it appears that we would be better off avoiding them.

Both the process of extracting polyunsaturated oils from plants or seeds and the process of creating partially hydrogenated products from them generate a significant proportion of trans fatty acids. Trans fatty acids raise LDL ("bad") cholesterol nearly as efficiently as saturated fats, but at least the saturated fats also raise the HDL ("good") cholesterol. Trans fatty acids do not. Furthermore, they may also raise triglyceride levels, so that some researchers consider them at least as much of a threat to health—if not more so—than saturated fats. How much trans fatty acid is too much? No one knows, and thus far no professional organization or government agency has suggested a specific daily limit. While completely eliminating trans fatty acids from your diet is neither practical nor necessary, limiting them is definitely a good idea. Indeed, in July 2003 the Food and Drug Administration (FDA) mandated that the amount of trans fatty acids in foods must be displayed on nutrition information labels by January 2006. (The FDA estimates that by 2009, reduced consumption of trans fatty acids resulting from food labeling, as well as voluntary efforts by manufacturers to reduce the amounts of these compounds in foods, will prevent 600 to 1,200 heart attacks and save 250 to 500 lives every year.)

Introducing some "good" fats—the essential fatty acids

There's one other important issue about the types of unsaturated fats that we eat. Our body is able to manufacture all of the fatty acids we need from other materials in our diet—carbohydrates, fats, and proteins—except for two, which have similar (and somewhat confusing) names: linoleic acid (abbreviated LA) and linolenic acid (abbreviated LNA). Because they must be taken directly from food sources, these are called essential fatty acids. From these two compounds, we make a number of other substances that play vital roles in immunity, the inflammatory response, clot formation, and the structure of cell membranes.

Based on its chemical structure, linoleic acid is called an omega-6 fatty acid, and it is relatively abundant in our food supply, occurring in seeds and any polyunsaturated oils made from them, corn and peanut oils, and animal fat (including poultry). Linolenic acid is called an omega-3 fatty acid and, unlike linoleic acid, is far less plentiful in our diet. It is found in flaxseed, walnuts, soybeans, canola, and their oils. It is also present in dark leafy green vegetables, though in lesser amounts.

Two omega-3 fatty acids with tongue-twisting names—eicosapentaenoic and docosahexaenoic acids, better known by their initials EPA and DHA—have been identified as particularly important to the well-being of the heart, blood vessels, and nervous system. DHA is also an important component of cell membranes in the brain, and both EPA and DHA are considered crucial to development of the brain (as well as that of the eye) before birth and during infancy. Some researchers have also been exploring the possibility that inadequate amounts of DHA play a role in the development of depression, schizophrenia, bipolar disorder, and other behavioral and neurological disturbances.

Our body can make EPA and DHA from linolenic acid in our diet—but there's a catch. First, many of us don't consume significant quantities of flaxseed, canola, walnuts, and soybeans on a daily basis—they're not exactly staples at the drive-through. In addition, the more omega-6 fatty acids in the diet, the less efficient is our production of the beneficial EPA and DHA from omega-3 fatty acids. In fact, some have raised concerns about the ratio of omega-6 to omega-3 fatty acids in the modern Western diet, proposing that an ideal diet would contain no more than four times as much omega-6 as omega-3.

A widely recommended response to the research supporting the benefits of omega-3 fatty acids is to add some to our diet in the form of fatty, cold-water fish—

salmon, mackerel, lake trout, albacore tuna, herring, and sardines. These contain the beneficial fatty acids EPA and DHA already formed and in more generous amounts than in their leaner counterparts, such as cod, orange roughy, sole, and flounder. While an ideal daily amount of omega-3 fatty acids has not been established, the American Heart Association recommends that the average adult have at least two servings of these fish every week, with some cautions for pregnant women.

People who are at high risk for coronary artery disease, or who already have it, should try to consume enough omega-3 fatty acids to include about a gram per day of EPA and DHA. This can usually be obtained from a three- to four-ounce serving of any of the cold-water fish just mentioned, but not everyone may be ready to eat fish every day. However, EPA and DHA can also be obtained in supplements that are usually derived from fish oils.

RECOMMENDATIONS FOR DAILY FAT INTAKE

The Institute of Medicine (IOM) recommends that 20 to 35 percent of total daily calories come from fat. For children, the percentage of total fat may be a little higher because of the need for fat in the developing central nervous system. Among children four to eighteen years of age, 25 to 35 percent of daily calories may come from fat; for one- to three-year-olds, 30 to 40 percent. The IOM has recommended that adult men obtain 17 grams and women 12 grams daily of linoleic acid, and 1.6 grams (men) and 1.1 grams (women) of linolenic acid daily. These are considered Adequate Intake (AI) levels, because Recommended Daily Allowances (RDAs) have yet to be determined. The IOM has not established specific guidelines regarding any other types of fats, but rather recommends simply that saturated fats, trans fats, and cholesterol be kept to a minimum.

Can I keep a good balance of fat in my diet?

1. Limit the saturated fat to 10 percent or less of your total daily calories. The current guidelines from prominent health research and advisory groups such as the American Heart Association and the American Dietetic Association typically recommend limiting saturated fats to 10 percent or less of total calories per day. For someone on a 2,000-calorie diet, this means that 600 calories would come from all fats combined (or about 65 grams of fat), and 200 calories (about 22 grams) from saturated fat.

   This is one situation in which the Nutrition Facts label displayed on many foods can be very helpful, since it lists not only the amount of saturated fat in the food, but also the percentage of the Daily Value (%DV)—that is, the percentage of the total day's allotment, assuming that you're trying to take no more than 10 percent of your total daily calories from saturated fat. (Keep in mind that most Nutrition Facts labels also assume that your total daily intake is either 2,000 or 2,500 calories.)

The most abundant sources of saturated fats are red meats, butter, ice cream, and other dairy products, as well as tropical (palm and coconut) oils. A mere tablespoon of butter, for example, contains 7 grams of saturated fat—about a third of the recommended daily amount for someone eating 2,000 calories per day. Coconut oil is 92 percent saturated fat, while 50 percent of palm oil is saturated fat. Some practical ways to keep the saturated fats at a reasonable level include:

- Limit your meat intake to about six ounces per day. Better yet, consider going "Mediterranean style" and eating red meat only a few times per month, and poultry and eggs only a few times per week.
- Choose leaner forms of beef. Avoid the marbled (fat-laden) cuts. Look for ground round containing lower percentages of fat—10 percent or less, if possible.
- Roasting, baking, grilling, broiling, and stir-frying meat are preferable to frying it.
- Trim the fat from your beef and pork, and remove the skin from your chicken.
- When you buy tuna or other meats in a can, you're better off choosing those that are packed in water. If you get oil-packed meats, rinse them in warm water to remove the fat.
- If you're drinking whole milk, try switching to milk

containing 2 percent fat. If you're used to 2 percent, try some one percent. If the watery texture isn't a turnoff, see how you do with nonfat. All of these forms are clearly marked in the dairy case.

- You can also try low-fat or nonfat versions of cheese, yogurt, sour cream, and ice cream.
- Try low-fat or nonfat versions of your favorite salad dressings. Remember, the regular forms can deliver more than 150 calories in two tablespoons.
- Before using butter (in whatever capacity), ask yourself whether olive oil would work just as well. It's a lot better for you.

2. Watch out for the trans fats. Foods that contain trans fatty acids (we'll call them "trans fats" for short) are pretty hard to avoid without subjecting your family to a rather spartan diet. But some that contain unhealthy portions of these compounds deserve to be reduced from your family's table, or eliminated altogether. The FDA estimates that the typical American adult consumes nearly 6 grams of trans fats every day. Some of this occurs naturally in animal products such as milk, cheese, butter, and red meats—the same foods that are rich in saturated fats. The vast majority, however, occurs in products containing naturally occurring fats that have been processed in some way, usually involving partial hydrogenation. These include:

- Stick margarine. This spread contains nearly 3 grams of trans fat per tablespoon (and 2 grams of saturated fat). By contrast, butter contains a mere 0.3 grams of trans fat, but more than 7 grams of saturated fat per tablespoon.

Some who have heard about the trans fat problem have dumped margarine and gone back to butter, but take note that tub margarine usually has much less of both trans and saturated fat. If you buy margarine, *read the labels* to find brands that have little or no trans fat.

- Baked goods. Perennial pleasures such as cakes, doughnuts, and cookies, aside from their sugar (and very often processed flour) content, are also likely to contain generous doses of trans fats. (A doughnut, for example, can pack 5 grams each of trans and saturated fat.) Ditto for packaged cake and baking mixes.
- Chips and crackers. A small bag of chips contains about 3 grams of trans fat. If it's fried or buttery in texture, you can assume trans fats are present.
- Frozen treats. Pizzas, pies, waffles, and breaded fish and chicken also contain trans fat.
- Fast foods. The primary offenders are fried chicken and french fries. Their last moments prior to entering your digestive tract are spent in frying in hydrogenated or partially hydrogenated oil. While in recent years many fast-food restaurants have cut back on their use of trans fat, a medium serving of fries can still contain a sizeable 4 or 5 grams of trans fat.

3. Keep an eye on the cholesterol content of foods. The USDA recommends that adults limit their daily intake of cholesterol to 300 mg or less. The American Heart Association repeats this recommendation for healthy adults and sets 200 mg, less than the amount in a single egg yolk, as the upper limit for individuals with cardiovascular disease or its risk factors. As we have already mentioned, the vast

majority of the cholesterol in our blood is generated by the liver, in amounts profoundly influenced by genetics and weight. Our daily intake of saturated and trans fats can also significantly affect blood cholesterol levels. The impact of the cholesterol that comes from our food, however, can be quite variable. For many people, eliminating or adding cholesterol in the diet has little impact on the amount circulating in the blood. For others, the effect is somewhat more significant. If you are trying to lower your cholesterol through dietary efforts, cutting back on saturated and trans fats will usually accomplish more than trying to limit cholesterol intake alone. Of course, a number of foods (such as red meats and cheese) contain generous amounts of both saturated fats and cholesterol, so limiting foods with saturated fats often will reduce the cholesterol as well.

Eggs, on the other hand, pose a nutritional dilemma. Each contains more than 200 mg of cholesterol (all of it in the yolk), but also some polyunsaturated fat, very little saturated fat (about 1.5 grams), and about 7 grams of high-quality protein. Thus far no research has shown a clear relationship between eating eggs on a regular basis and developing coronary artery disease, and one could argue that an egg cooked using a little vegetable oil represents a more nutritious breakfast option than a doughnut full of trans fats or a few slices of white toast. Of course, eating the egg white without the yolk will eliminate the cholesterol, as will using a no-cholesterol egg substitute.

4. Get enough of the "good" fats. Earlier in this chapter we explained why monounsaturated fatty acids, especially the omega-6 and omega-3 fatty acids, are beneficial to life and health. We also mentioned some good sources for these beneficial fats, and we'll recap them here:

- Become a regular user of olive oil, which contains more than 70 percent monounsaturated fatty acids. Buy the extra virgin oil, which comes from the first pressing of the fruit. Among other things, you can dip bread in it (rather than using butter) and use it when you stir-fry or sauté vegetables or meat. When not in use, keep it in a dark cupboard.

- If you don't care for olive oil, try other vegetable oils that contain high percentages of monounsaturated fatty acids, including canola, peanut, and soybean oils. You may find canola oil more to your liking for baking than olive oil.

- Eat at least two servings of fish per week.

- Try adding flaxseed to a variety of foods or as an ingredient in baking.

- Add nuts and seeds to your diet, especially as a substitute for less healthy snacks such as chips, or even as a source of protein. An ounce of nuts, for example, contains 8 grams of protein, roughly the same amount as in a glass of milk. Watch out, however, because these are calorie-dense foods—an ounce of walnuts contains 160 calories—and it's easy to down a bowlful without realizing that you've just swallowed several hundred calories. Depending upon their preparation, they also may have a fair amount of salt or sugar. Think *handfuls*: a serving size is an ounce; for example, roughly fifteen to twenty cashews.

- Try avocado slices instead of cheese on your sandwiches.

6

CHOOSE SUPPLEMENTS CAREFULLY

Did you chew (or gag) on a vitamin pill every day when you were growing up, cheered on by Mom's pronouncements that it would "help you grow big and strong"? Do you become glassy-eyed in the aisle at the supermarket where battalions of vitamins, minerals, and other supplements line the shelves? Do you wonder whether you can get all the vitamins you need from a bowl of fortified cereal, or if you need to spend a small fortune every month on a tackle box of supplements?

You've probably gotten an earful of advice on this subject from just about every direction—except one. If you haven't heard much from your doctor about vitamin and mineral supplements, you're not alone. Professional organizations and physicians have generally taken the "food is enough" approach: If you're a healthy individual consistently eating three square meals a day, all of the vitamins and minerals necessary for good health should be available on your plate. Taking a lot of supplements wastes money and may even risk toxicity.

Other voices argue that our food isn't as good as it used to be in the good old days: Modern technology, processing, and pollutants, the stresses of life, and fast-food eating habits have all conspired to downgrade what's on our daily table, so every day we need to take a comprehensive vitamin/mineral tablet or elixir, and perhaps a whole assortment of supplements, to stay healthy.

Which of these positions is right? To get a handle on this question, we'll need a little background information about these substances.

WHAT ARE VITAMINS?

Vitamins are nutrients with the following characteristics:

- They are essential, in that they are vital to health, even life itself. In addition, the term *essential* in nutritional vocabulary means that *they cannot be created within the body from other nutrients* but must be obtained from food (or supplements). An exception to the second meaning of *essential* is vitamin D, which for its synthesis requires a modest amount of sun exposure. (Without adequate sun exposure, vitamin D must be supplied from food or supplements.)
- They are organic—that is, they contain carbon (as opposed to minerals, which are *inorganic*).
- They are *needed only in tiny amounts*, and thus are micronutrients. Daily requirements for vitamins are

measured in milligrams (mg) or micrograms (mcg), as opposed to grams or ounces, which are used for macronutrients—carbohydrates, fats, and proteins.

• Vitamins *do not serve as fuel* (they are not broken down to create energy), nor do they form any structures. Instead, most of them participate in important biochemical reactions.

During the first half of the twentieth century, thirteen compounds were identified as vitamins. Since 1948, when vitamin B_{12} was isolated, no new vitamins have been discovered. (Several compounds have been proposed as vitamins, but none have incontrovertibly met the scientific criteria to be designated as one.) The thirteen well-identified vitamins are divided into two groups:

1. The eight B vitamins (also called the B complex) and vitamin C. These vitamins, with the exception of vitamin B_{12}, are not stored for long periods of time, so regular replenishment from food or supplements every few days (if not more often) is necessary to maintain health.

2. Vitamins A, D, E, and K. Excess amounts of these vitamins are stored in fat and the liver rather than being excreted by the kidneys—a useful process if there is an extended dietary shortage, because these vitamins may then be available even if none are taken in food for weeks or even months. But if very large doses are taken on a regular basis, toxicity may occur. (As with any nutrient, there is always the possibility of too much of a good thing.)

WHAT ARE MINERALS?

We need a steady supply of certain minerals to stay healthy. In the realm of nutrition, minerals are distinct from vitamins in some important ways. Minerals are inorganic (so don't let anyone try to sell you "organic" minerals); unlike vitamins, they cannot be broken down or destroyed by exposure to light or heat. All vitamins are micronutrients—present and needed in the body in very small amounts—but minerals are divided into two categories based on the quantities we need. Major minerals are present in the body in amounts totaling more than 5 grams. These include calcium, phosphorus, potassium, sulfur, sodium, chloride, and magnesium. Trace or micro minerals, on the other hand, weigh in at well under 5 grams in a normal adult, and they are needed in quantities measured in milligrams or even micrograms. They are no less important, however. Trace minerals include iron, zinc, copper, manganese, iodine, selenium, fluoride, chromium, and molybdenum.

Unlike many of the vitamins (especially the B complex and C), with trace minerals and magnesium *there is a narrow margin between amounts that are needed for normal function and amounts that are toxic*. Therefore, it is especially desirable to obtain these substances from foods if at all possible. If you use supplements for trace minerals, you should avoid taking more than 100 percent of the recommended daily allowance (RDA) on an ongoing basis.

WHAT ARE ANTIOXIDANTS?

Over the past several years, attaching the word *antioxidant* to any product has become a buzzword meaning "It's good for you, no matter what the problem," much like the words *natural* or *organic* in previous decades. What exactly are antioxidants, and what do they do for us?

While a steady supply of oxygen is necessary for basic metabolic operations in every cell, oxygen's reactions with a variety of compounds can generate highly unstable molecules called free radicals. Free radicals can damage other molecules, including fatty acids, proteins, and even DNA, the molecule that serves as the genetic blueprint for the cell. A number of enzymes inactivate free radicals. With the passage of time, however, these may become less effective or may simply be overwhelmed. Coming to the aid of our cells are the antioxidants, substances (such as vitamins C and E) that work to stabilize free radicals and prevent them from damaging other molecules. Certain minerals— notably selenium, manganese, copper, and zinc—while not antioxidants themselves, are necessary for the proper function of antioxidant enzymes.

A growing body of research suggests links between diets rich in antioxidants and lower rates of coronary artery disease, cancer, and cataracts and macular degeneration. So it follows that taking generous amounts of them in supplements should seriously improve one's health and well-being—right? For years a multi-billion-dollar supplement industry has been shouting "Amen!" all the way to the bank, but hard data to back its enthusiastic claims has been difficult to come by. One notorious example: Beta-carotene, an antioxidant found in deeply pigmented fruits and vegetables, appeared to be a prime candidate for supplement superstardom. But four large randomized controlled studies comparing the health of people who were given a beta-carotene supplement with that of an equal number of people given an identical-appearing placebo (with no biological effect) revealed little difference between the effects of the two. Other studies have had similar results. The important lesson here is that taking supplements containing antioxidants is no substitute for consuming them in foods.

SHOULD I TAKE A VITAMIN/MINERAL SUPPLEMENT?

Even in our well-fed society, certain groups of people may be vulnerable to one or more shortfalls in vitamins or minerals. These include people who are unable to obtain, prepare, swallow, or absorb an adequate supply of basic nutrients because of:

- Chronic illness, especially when it affects appetite or the absorption of food
- Poverty
- Alcoholism or other drug addiction

- Major psychological or emotional problems—especially schizophrenia, significant depression, or other behavioral problems, including eating disorders

Along with these more extreme situations, a number of people do not consume a balanced or adequate diet every day. Others might need an extra supply of one or more nutrients because of a special situation:

- The elderly, who may have to cope with chronic illness, multiple medications, depression, memory problems, and loss of mobility. Seniors who are living alone may develop erratic eating habits, and some may battle alcoholism.
- Dieters, especially those on weight-loss plans that banish entire groups of foods (such as very strict low-carbohydrate or low-fat approaches). A variation on this theme is the picky eater, young or old, who sticks to a narrow repertoire of foods.
- Fast-food addicts, especially those whose primary source of fruits and vegetables is whatever is found between the burger and the bun.
- Adolescents, who not only may frequently eat fast-food meals but also may have erratic eating habits (such as skipping breakfast before running off to school). Furthermore, their rapid growth and development requires a steady supply of high-quality nutrients.
- Smokers, whose habit depletes the body of vitamin C.
- Strict vegetarians (vegans) who consume no animal products of any kind.
- People recovering from surgery, a major injury, or a burn.
- Women who are pregnant or breast-feeding (or who may become pregnant).

- Women with heavy, lengthy, or more frequent menstrual periods, who are at risk for iron deficiency.

Despite the dire warnings of many would-be nutritional experts (who more often than not have some expensive products to sell), it is not necessary to take handfuls of supplements to remain healthy. Nevertheless, a number of reputable, conservative researchers and organizations consider a daily multivitamin and mineral supplement to be a good investment—especially for someone who falls into one of the categories listed above.

HOW DO I CHOOSE A VITAMIN/ MINERAL SUPPLEMENT?

1. Think of a supplement as a safety net. They should serve as nutritional insurance—not as a quick way to get around making good food choices. Putting an additive in your gas tank can't substitute for poor-quality fuel or no fuel at all.

2. Look for a comprehensive supplement. It should supply 100 percent of the daily value (DV) for most of the thirteen vitamins and the trace minerals we have mentioned in this chapter. In particular, look for 100 percent daily value for the B vitamins (including folic acid), C, D, E, iron, iodine, zinc, selenium, copper, manganese, chromium, and molybdenum.

3. Beware of inflated prices. Your comprehensive sup-

plement should be inexpensive—no more than ten to twenty cents per day. If you're shelling out thirty dollars or more every month for vitamins and minerals, you're spending too much. Pick a less expensive brand and spend the difference at the produce section or a local vegetable stand.

4. Beware of inflated doses. Taking up to 200 percent of the Daily Value for the B vitamins won't hurt you, but unless you have specific directions from a physician to use high doses of other vitamins and minerals, think carefully before buying a megadose preparation. (Two exceptions are vitamins C and E, which we will discuss momentarily.) Vitamin A and many of the minerals can be toxic in large doses.

5. Beware of inflated claims. Many advertisements and infomercials claim that a concoction has special, unique, all-natural, superpotent, stress-reducing, life-extending, youth-restoring, energy-boosting, cosmic, good-for-what-ails-ya ingredients and additives. They want $29.99 or more per month, usually with a special offer if you call right now ("Operators are waiting!"). If you suspect that it sounds too good to be true, you'll be correct 99.9 percent of the time.

6. Look for the letters USP on the label. This indicates that the product meets the standards of the United States Pharmacopeia (USP), a nonprofit, nongovernmental organization that sets manufacturing

standards for drugs, supplements, and other health-care products.

7. Better yet, look for a logo that says "USP-Verified Dietary Supplement." This indicates that the product has undergone more rigorous voluntary testing for verification of ingredients, good manufacturing procedures, absence of contaminants, and dissolving characteristics (to ensure that it can be absorbed effectively once swallowed). Products that have passed this muster are also checked over time using random samples from store shelves. A current list of verified supplements can be found at http://www.usp.org/USPVerified/.

8. Don't worry about getting 100 percent of the Daily Value for phosphorus, potassium, chloride, biotin, or vitamin K from your multivitamin. These typically appear as low percent DVs on multivitamins because you get the vast majority from your food. (The current RDA for biotin, 30 mcg, is now 10 percent of the amount used in estimating the DV.) If you are low in potassium, your doctor will prescribe an appropriate preparation and follow your progress with blood tests.

9. You don't need to use a liquid supplement unless you can't swallow tablets. Some liquid supplements are marketed with the claim that vitamins and minerals are better absorbed in liquid form than from tablets. This may indeed be true—if the tablet doesn't disintegrate.

USP recommends that a vitamin tablet disintegrate completely thirty to forty-five minutes after being swallowed, another reason to seek brands that meet USP standards. Unfortunately, claims that liquid vitamins are uniformly superior to tablets originate from marketers and not from professional organizations. Similarly, some notoriously misleading advertisements for "colloidal" liquid mineral preparations have been in circulation on cassette tapes and the Internet for years. Assuming you can swallow a good-quality tablet, there is no reason to pay inflated prices for a liquid formulation.

10. Keep all vitamin and mineral preparations in a safe place where children cannot find and accidentally swallow them. Remember that the amount of iron in a few adult multivitamin/mineral tablets can be lethal to a small child.

In addition to using a single comprehensive supplement as a nutritional safety net, you may want to consider some additional vitamins and minerals for your daily routine:

- Additional vitamin C (250 to 500 mg) and vitamin E (200 IU). These are doses at which you may obtain antioxidant benefits from these two vitamins. Recent research suggests that daily doses of 500 mg of vitamin C and 400 international units (IU) of vitamin E on an ongoing basis may reduce the risk of developing Alzheimer's disease. But analysis of multiple studies has raised concern that ongoing vitamin E doses of 400

IU or more may be associated with higher rates of death from all causes. The jury is still out, but you may obtain some overall benefit and are probably safe in taking 250 to 500 mg of vitamin C and 200 IU of vitamin E daily. These quantities are not found in typical multivitamin tablets, and while it's possible to take in this much vitamin C from food sources, there is no way to obtain this much vitamin E from food. Remember that if you are a smoker, you need more vitamin C.

- Additional calcium. Because calcium is so bulky, most multivitamins contain only 100 to 200 mg. The recommended daily allowance for adults ranges from 1,000 to 1,300 mg, with many experts suggesting 1,500 mg for women after menopause. Because calcium intake from food may vary, many adults should add a calcium supplement, with or without vitamin D.

- Additional iron and folic acid if you are pregnant. The RDA for iron during pregnancy is 27 mg, while a typical multivitamin contains 18 mg. Similarly, the RDA for folic acid during pregnancy is 600 mcg, while most multivitamins contain 400 mcg. Rather than looking for additional iron and folic acid tablets, however, your best bet would be to use prenatal vitamins prescribed by your physician, which usually contain 1,000 mcg of folic acid and 25 to 30 mg of iron.

While vitamins and other supplements can be beneficial (and for some, even lifesaving), *they are not a substitute for wise food choices*. As clever as we might become through research and development of nutritional products, no one can duplicate the rich and complex blend of nutrients in food, especially fruits and vegetables. Remember, the only truly natural products are found in the produce section of the supermarket. An important corollary: Supplements cannot compensate for a lifetime of poor lifestyle choices (smoking, overeating, abusing drugs and alcohol, refusing to exercise, and so forth).

7

TRACK YOUR EATING PATTERNS

By now you may have asked a very important question: How do I translate all of these recommendations into actual decisions about the kinds of foods that I buy, prepare, order at a restaurant, and ultimately eat? How many of us actually calculate, or even have a rough idea, what percentage of our daily calories come from carbohydrates, fats, and fiber? And do these percentages tell the whole story of our nutritional health?

We could, of course, shrug our shoulders and proceed with business as usual: eat what and however much we like, guided by family traditions, taste buds, emotions, advertising, and convenience. In the United States, however, that approach has led to an epidemic of obesity and contributed to an increase in cardiovascular disease and diabetes. (Some cancers and a number of other chronic diseases may also be the by-product of this approach.) If we want to take some positive, proactive steps toward improving our personal and family fuel, how might we proceed? Here are several ideas.

READ THE NUTRITION FACTS LABEL

In the United States, the Food and Drug Administration (FDA) requires that packaged foods bear a Nutrition Facts label that includes pertinent information about what's inside. Even if you don't keep a running

Nutrition Facts

Serving Size 1 Cup (228g)
Serving Per Container 2

Amount Per Serving

Calories 100	Calories from Fat 10

	% Daily Value*
Total Fat 3g*	**5%**
Saturated Fat 1g	**5%**
Trans Fat 1.5g	
Cholesterol 0mg	**0%**
Sodium 188mg	**5%**
Total Carbohydrate 45g	**15%**
Dietary Fiber 4g	**16%**
Soluble Fiber 1g	
Sugars 20g	
Other Carbohydrates 21g	
Protein 5g	

Vitamin A	20%
Vitamin C	8%
Calcium	4%
Iron	15%
Vitamin D	20%
Vitamin E	25%
Thiamin	25%
Riboflavin	25%
Niacin	25%
Vitamin B6	100%
Folate	100%

tally of your daily nutrient intake, you should pay attention to at least some of the information on the label.

Highlights include:

Serving size. This number is important, since all of the facts on the label are based on a serving size that the label assumes you will eat. The serving size may be obvious (such as the entire can of soda) or less so. For example, the serving size for dry cereal is typically listed as one cup, which may be a bit less than you pour into the bowl every morning. The label on a container of crackers or chips will list a certain number of these as a serving—but do we ever keep count when we're enjoying one of these snacks? Serving sizes for salad dressings are usually two tablespoons, but you may be surprised how that compares to your typical dollop on that bowl of greens. Measuring the amount of the serving size—and the amount you actually use— for a number of your favorite foods can be an eye-opening experience.

Calories per serving. All of the numbers on the label must be adjusted if you use more or less than the stated serving size. The total number of calories you need every day depends on several factors: your age, gender, height, weight, activity level, and to some degree genetics (which affects the efficiency of your individual metabolic engine). In general, follow these approximate daily calorie goals:

- For children between two and six, some older adults, and many women: 1,600 calories.
- For the "average adult": 2,000 calories. On nutrition labels you will typically see 2,000 listed as the total number of daily calories.
- For older children, teenage girls, and active women: 2,200 calories.
- For teenage boys and active men: 2,800 calories.

Calories from fat. Divide this number by the calories per serving and multiply by 100. You'll get the percentage of calories derived from fat, which may or may not be useful, depending on the type of food. The fact that this number is included on the label is a reflection of the "fat is bad" doctrine that we have heard for decades. But the percentage of a food's calories derived from fat does not necessarily reflect its quality. Extra virgin olive oil is 100 percent fat, but it contains monounsaturated fatty acids that are beneficial to health.

Total fat, cholesterol, and quantities of saturated, monounsaturated, and polyunsaturated fats, which are more useful numbers. (Remember that trans fats are going to show up on labels as well.) These are listed in grams, and—for total fat, saturated fat, and cholesterol—as a percent daily value. The percent daily value (or %DV) is *not* the percent of calories in the serving, or the percent of total calories for the day, for fat or saturated fat in the serving. Instead, it is the percent of the maximum recommended amount of these substances for a person eating two thousand calories per day. This number is intended to help you get a handle on how much of a contribution the particular food is making to what should be your daily maximum. At the bottom of the Nutrition Facts label is a listing of these recommendations, under a statement that begins "Percent Daily Values are based on a 2,000-calorie diet." Most labels include not only the recommendations for 2,000 calories but for 2,500 as well. If your calorie target is much more or less than 2,000, the %DV for the particular food will be less or more than the amount on the label. The %DV listings are based on the assumption that we should keep our fat calories below a maximum of 25 percent and our saturated fats below 10 percent of the total number of calories we consume every day. For cholesterol, the assumption is that we should eat foods containing a total of 300 mg or less per day. Note that you will not find any %DV listings for mono-unsaturated or polyunsaturated fats. This means that the FDA hasn't provided recommended daily intakes for these nutrients.

Total carbohydrate, dietary fiber, and sugars. Of these, the most useful are the grams of fiber and sugars, since you want to get enough of the first and limit your intake of the second.

Protein. The Nutrition Facts label includes grams of protein per serving, but without an estimate of the percent daily value, because the recommended amount for an individual is based on his or her weight.

Other nutrients. The amounts of vitamins and minerals contained in a serving of the food are listed under the main nutrients.

Few people are going to work through the laborious process of calculating the daily percentages of their various nutrients, a task that can be even more challenging if you are actually *cooking*—combining various ingredients to create a masterpiece in the kitchen—as opposed to eating prepackaged food. Nevertheless, you should know your way around the Nutrition Facts label, because several of its statistics can help you make informed choices.

What do those phrases on the food label mean?

When the label on a food package says "low fat" or "good source of dietary fiber" or even "light," is that just an advertising gimmick to get your attention or does it actually mean something? As it turns out, the Food and Drug Administration (FDA) has spelled out specific guidelines for the various terms that you see when you browse the shelves at the supermarket. Here are some that may sound familiar:

No calories: Fewer than 5 calories per serving.

Low calorie, light, or lite in calories: Fewer than 40 calories per serving. For a meal or main dish, fewer than 120 calories per 100 grams (about three and a half ounces).

Fat-free or nonfat: Less than 0.5 gram of fat per serving.

Low fat, light, or lite in fat: Fewer than 3 grams of fat per serving. For a meal or main dish, fewer than 3 grams of fat per 100 grams, or less than 30 percent fat.

Saturated fat–free: Less than 0.5 gram of saturated fat per serving.

Low in saturated fat: Less than one gram of saturated fat and less than 15 percent of total calories from saturated fat per serving. For a meal or main dish, less than one gram of saturated fat per 100 grams or less than 10 percent saturated fat.

Cholesterol-free: Contains fewer than 2 milligrams of cholesterol per serving and 2 grams or fewer of saturated fat per serving.

Low in cholesterol: Fewer than 20 milligrams of cholesterol and 2 grams or less of saturated fat per serving.

Sugar-free: Less than 0.5 gram of sugar per serving.

No added sugar: No sugar or sugar-containing ingredient added during processing. (Not necessarily sugar-free, however, if the product naturally contains sugars.)

Reduced (less) calorie, fat, saturated fat, cholesterol, or sugar: At least 25 percent less of the particular substance than the same portion of a comparable product.

High fiber: Provides 5 grams or more of fiber per serving.

Good source of . . . : Provides 10 to 19 percent of the
Daily Value of the specific nutrient per serving.

High in . . . : Provides 20 percent or more of the Daily
Value of the specific nutrient per serving.

Lean (for meat and poultry products): Contains
fewer than 10 grams of fat, 4.5 grams of saturated
fat, and 95 grams of cholesterol per serving.

Extra lean: Contains fewer than 5 grams of fat, 2
grams of saturated fat, and 95 milligrams of cholesterol per serving.

FOLLOW THE FOOD GUIDE PYRAMID

You may remember hearing or learning in school about
the Food Guide Pyramid—a diagram created by the
United States Department of Agriculture (USDA) and
the United States Department of Health and Human
Services that combined foods into various groups and
then recommended that we eat a certain number of
servings from each group each day. The base of the
pyramid was occupied by the bread, cereal, rice, and
pasta group because the USDA recommended six to
eleven servings of foods from it every day. Vegetables,
with three to five servings per day, shared the next level
with fruits (two to four servings). The next level was
shared by the milk and the meat groups, each with two
to three daily servings. At the apex of the pyramid sat
fats, oils, and sweets—not really food groups, but
rather the foods we were advised to "use sparingly."

With the publication of the 2005 edition of the *Dietary Guidelines for Americans*, the Food Guide Pyramid got a major overhaul. The "layers" of the pyramid, representing five basic food groups—grains, vegetables, fruits, milk, and meat and beans—have been flipped to a vertical orientation on the new pyramid, and they only vaguely suggest that some groups might be emphasized over others. Indeed, the pyramid offers virtually no nutritional information, but rather serves mainly as a symbol for the revised contents of the Dietary Guidelines and the new interactive Web site, http://www.mypyramid.gov, that supports it.

Unlike the original Food Guide Pyramid, the new version promotes exercise, emphasizes the benefits of whole grains, and makes an appropriate distinction between the healthier monounsaturated and polyunsaturated fats and the less healthy saturated and trans fats. Overall, the interactive Web site is a definite improvement over the old pyramid, provided one has access to a computer and the Internet. Those without these electronic tools can obtain a copy of the 2005 *Dietary Guidelines for Americans* by calling the U.S. Government Printing Office toll-free at (866) 512-1800.

ORIENT YOUR EATING HABITS AROUND SOME HEALTHY PRINCIPLES

So far this book has concentrated on the *kinds* of food we should be eating in order to maintain a healthy,

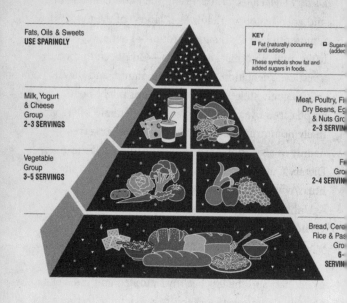

Fats, Oils & Sweets
USE SPARINGLY

KEY
⊡ Fat (naturally occurring and added)   ▨ Sugars (added)
These symbols show fat and added sugars in foods.

Milk, Yogurt & Cheese Group
2-3 SERVINGS

Meat, Poultry, Fi
Dry Beans, Eg
& Nuts Gro
2-3 SERVIN

Vegetable Group
3-5 SERVINGS

F
Gro
2-4 SERVIN

Bread, Cere
Rice & Pas
Gro
**6-
SERVIN**

Food pyramids created by the U.S. Department of Agriculture and the U.S. Department of Health and Human Ser

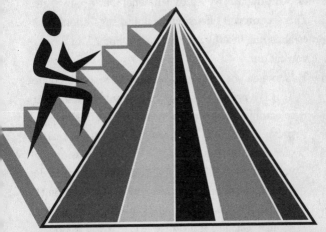

MyPyramid.gov
STEPS TO A HEALTHIER YOU

The 2005 Food Pyramid is designed to be an interactive tool that provides nutrition guidelines based on a person's age, gender, and level of physical activity. (To generate your own guidelines, visit http://www.mypyramid.gov.) The vertical shaded portions (from left to right) in the pyramid represent grains, vegetables, fruits, milk, and meat and beans.

well-balanced diet. But there are some other principles that are just as important for healthy eating that have to do with the *way* we eat (when, where, how much, etc.). This section will offer some practical suggestions for establishing healthy eating habits at home and when you eat out.

1. Eat when you're hungry—and stop when you're not. This is a profoundly simple idea, but we're so used to eating for every possible reason that this may prove harder than it sounds. Before you start eating, or before the next bite, get in the habit of asking yourself, *Am I (still) hungry?* You may be surprised at how often the answer is *Not really,* at which point you need to ask, *So why am I reaching for something to put in my mouth?* If the answer is that you're upset, bored, or trying to relax, then ask yourself if there are other ways to solve that problem, even if they may not seem as quick and effective as your favorite food. If the answer is, *I'm enjoying this, and I don't feel like stopping,* then at least slow down. Here's a news flash—you're more likely to yield to the worst food temptations if you're famished. If you're actually feeling hungry, you should eat something—but of course *what* and *how much* will be the critical issues.

   By the way, most of us eat so often that we don't know the difference between real hunger and every other vague uneasiness that seems to respond to food. If you have any doubt, try skipping one or two meals and note how you feel. Then as an experiment, see how little food it takes to end that sensation.

2. Stop eating when you're satisfied, but before you're really full. We all enjoy eating a traditional Thanksgiving dinner, but how often have you left the table feeling more stuffed than the turkey? That bloated, heavy, drowsy sensation really isn't very pleasant, nor are the heartburn and gas that may join the party a little later. Unfortunately, eating a complete dinner at many restaurants—or perhaps at your dining-room table—will bring on the same sensation. In many cultures children are taught to stop eating before they feel full, and we should learn to do likewise. (Hunger will be gone long before you've eaten half of the amount that brings fullness.)

3. Eat slowly. If you've ever been interrupted for several minutes after the first few bites of a meal, you may have noticed that you weren't particularly hungry when you sat down again. This is a very important validation of the fact that *whether we eat quickly or slowly, hunger goes away in about the same amount of time*. Think of it another way. After you begin eating, it takes about fifteen to twenty minutes for signals from the stomach and changes in blood glucose to signal that you're no longer hungry. If you are inhaling your food during that time, you can put away

hundreds of calories—and yet be no more satisfied than if you took a fraction of that amount.

If you really enjoy food, eating slowly is the only way to go:

- Put down your utensils between bites.
- After cutting a piece of meat, put the knife down and pick up the fork with the hand that held the knife—then eat the piece of meat. (This avoids the rapid-fire fork-to-mouth routine.)
- Take smaller bites.
- Thoroughly chew, and savor the taste and texture of each mouthful.
- Pause between bites. If you're with others, enjoy the conversation. If everyone is too busy eating to talk, start some conversation so that *they'll* slow down. (If a TV is the yammering "guest" at your meal, by all means turn it off.) A shared meal at which no one is talking is a wasted opportunity. If you're eating alone, stop and give thanks for every bite.

4. Think differently about portions (part 1). Forget about sixteen-ounce steaks and baked potatoes the size of a football. Think instead about adopting some of the following portion sizes—none of which require you to use a food scale—for foods that are often sources of runaway calories:

- A piece of lean meat the size of a deck of cards
- A potato the size of a small lightbulb
- A serving of cheese the size of one or two pairs of dice
- A serving of butter the size of one of those dice
- A serving of pasta the size of a computer mouse
- A one-cup serving of cereal (one of the good kinds,

without all of the added sugar), which is also the amount in one of those individual-sized boxes
- One slice of bread, half a bagel, half an English muffin, or half a bun

Notice that we didn't list serving sizes for foods like broccoli, apples, and celery sticks. The vast majority of vegetables and fruits are part of the solution to healthy eating rather than part of the problem, unless they're swimming in rich sauces or syrups.

5. Think differently about portions (part 2).
   - Instead of the typical dinner plate, use a salad plate to hold your usual fare. (You can have another salad plate for the salad.)
   - Don't eat any more than you can fit on that plate—no stacking allowed—and no going back for seconds.
   - Take your sweet time eating your meal.

Remember the good old days when you would receive an actual hot meal on a long airline flight? Remember the tiny salad and the little rectangular container that held the main course? There wasn't much there, but because it filled the dish completely it always seemed like enough food. If you're trying to reduce portions and place some smaller servings on your old dinner plate, all of that open space may look alarming. *Is that all I get??* Put it on a smaller plate, however, and your brain will adjust its perception and your emotions.

6. Think differently about portions (part 3). Here's the simplest, cheapest, most surefire weight-loss

program on the planet, and it involves only three basic steps:

- Put whatever you're used to eating at a given meal on your plate.
- Take half of it away.
- Eat what remains slowly enough to last as long as your regular portions.

Okay, so this advice was a little tongue-in-cheek, but not entirely. Removing half of your usual portions would be a pretty drastic change, but it would certainly help you to think about how much food you really need and keep you from gaining unwanted pounds. Taking away a quarter or a third of your typical portions will almost certainly accomplish the same thing over time, assuming you stick with it.

7. Avoid random or nonpurposeful eating. There are all sorts of occasions when we eat not because we're hungry or even to comfort ourselves (more on that later), but just because the food happens to appear before us. A lot of people have trouble with this at the workplace: Someone has a birthday or a coworker brings leftovers from a party at home, and suddenly there's an array of our favorite snack foods on the counter as we pass by. If it's something we like, it's all too easy to reach for it without thinking, an automatic reflex between brain, arm, and mouth. It takes some effort, but it's critical to ask yourself the all-important questions: (1) *Am I actually hungry?*

(2) If I am actually hungry, is this plateful of cake/cookies/chips the best way to relieve my hunger?

If you're an autopilot eater, you must create an environment at home that reduces the likelihood of this behavior. It's very simple: When you're done eating, put *all* of the food away. You can consider making an exception for a bowl of fruit, especially if you're trying to reprogram your household to enjoy more nutritious snacks. Some important variations on this theme:

- The big one: eating in front of the TV. While engrossed in a program or a movie you can easily lose track of what you're eating and consume a tremendous quantity of food. Plus, you're likely to see enticing ads for all kinds of food. If there's going to be food in the TV room, *you* decide ahead of time what and how much. Don't just bring boxes, bags, and bowls of stuff to graze on.

- Eating at sporting events and movies. For many sports fans and moviegoers, a nonstop flow of food has become a necessary part of the show. The same can be true, of course, during a busy weekend of games on TV or a movie fest at home. Once again a little planning can save you hundreds of excess calories, not to mention a wad of cash. For one thing, don't come to the game or movie hungry. If the venue allows it, bring some healthier snacks of your own, such as fruit or sticks of carrots or celery. If not, look for smaller sizes or split larger quantities among two or more people. Consider getting ice water instead of a soft drink, and hold the butter on the popcorn. And as always, ask the important question: *Am I still hungry?*

- Eating during other activities. When at home, eat only from one (modest-sized) plate, in one room, doing absolutely nothing else. If you want a snack, fine—just measure out a reasonable portion on your special plate, and then eat it at your kitchen or dining-room table without watching TV, reading, studying, or doing anything else. (Obviously, having a conversation with another person is okay—otherwise, eating becomes like sharing a trough in the barn.) In general this is a good idea for limiting random, unconscious eating, but with one exception. If you're eating an actual meal (as opposed to a snack) by yourself, reading may help you *take your time* with it, as long as you keep track of your hunger/fullness status.

8. Get comfortable leaving food behind. Many of us are driven by the insane notion that we are obliged to finish whatever food appears on our plate. This may arise from exhortations during childhood to "Join the clean-plate club" or "Remember that people are starving in Africa," or messages from Mom or Grandma that preparing food is a gesture of love and eating it is a way of saying thank you. How many times have we kept eating (especially in a restaurant and often long after being full) because we didn't want food to go to waste? If the only two destinations for that food are the trash bin or the bulging fat stores in our body, which is the better place for it

to go? "I paid good money for that food," you might protest. But what is the excess fat costing you? And if you're in a restaurant, your server will gladly give you a box or bag to take home the extra for another day.

Very important parenting tip: Don't encourage or exhort kids to eat when they're not hungry, and don't threaten to punish them for not cleaning their plates. There are much healthier ways to influence what they eat.

9. Be very careful when you eat out. Enjoying restaurant meals can be both a treat and a trap. Yes, it's nice for special occasions, but all too often we opt for the drive-through, the pizza delivery, or even a complete sit-down meal because we're too rushed or hassled or tired to prepare food ourselves. About 25 percent of American meals are not home cooked, and that's not counting "nuke and serve" foods from the freezer. Not only can this be a drain on the pocketbook, but many restaurants serve up very large portions, whether or not they're designated as supersized. Here are some suggestions to help draw the line between dining out and pigging out:

- Try to avoid bringing a ravenous appetite to the restaurant. You'll be tempted to order more items than you really need.
- Take your time. The fact that families often go to restaurants because there isn't time to *prepare* a meal doesn't mean that "eating out" has to mean "eat and

run." The best restaurant experiences are those in which the meal is an occasion to share good conversation, not to rush through the food. The more expensive fine-dining establishments have this figured out: They tend to serve smaller portions (often exquisitely prepared) at a leisurely pace, leaving you satisfied but not bloated.

- Split entrees. If you and your companion can find something you both like, this will save both money and calories.
- As we just said, you don't have to clean your plate. Stop when you're pleasantly satisfied, and ask to have what remains put in a container to take home.
- Skip dessert or order one for the whole table to share.
- Stay out of fast-food restaurants. The products they serve are carefully engineered to be highly satisfying—indeed, some would argue that they are addictive, especially to young palates whose business they aggressively court. In response to rising criticism about dispensing nutritional junk, the fast-food industry has started to offer some alternatives to the usual burgers and fries, including salads, broiled chicken entrées, and fruit. But their staple items remain highly processed, calorie dense, and loaded with saturated fat, salt, and sugar.
- If you can't stay out of fast-food restaurants, skip the fries and look for a salad. Avoid supersizing, the marketing ploy that seems like such a bargain but packs huge amounts of extra calories. The only items that get supersized are fries and soft drinks, which you should avoid anyway. Get the kids—and yourselves—milk or water instead of a soft drink.

- Avoid buffets, or at least don't come with a huge appetite. When faced with a buffet meal, follow some of the other guidelines in this section: Put your choices on a smaller plate (usually the salad plate), eat slowly, quit before you're full, and don't feel obliged to finish what's on your plate, even though you put it there yourself.

10. Keep your eyes open for other ideas like these, and for recipes that utilize healthier foods and portions. No single source of advice, including this book, will address *every* issue you might have related to healthy eating or portions. While you don't want to obsess about what you eat or make food the center of your emotional universe, this is such an important topic that you would be wise to become a lifelong learner.

THE IMPORTANCE OF BREAKING BREAD TOGETHER

Before we conclude our look at healthy eating habits, we need a reminder about the importance of the *context* of our nourishment. We are not animals that graze in a field or gather at a trough. We are meant to be nourished at the table in more ways than merely transporting food from plate to stomach. Meals are a time for socializing, conversing, sharing, and celebrating.

Family meals can be particularly powerful events in the lives of both children and adults. They can and should be the occasion to share the day's events, decompress, commiserate, encourage one another, laugh, learn how to speak and listen politely, instill values, establish each person's identity as a member of a family, welcome guests, and acknowledge God's provision on a daily basis. They are, unfortunately, an endangered species, threatened by overcommitment, crowded calendars, and electronic distractions such as

TVs and phones. If you take away nothing else from this book, make a decision that shared family meals will become a priority in your home. As part of that process, consider the following:

- Set aside three, if not more, occasions per week for family meals. The expectation is that all hands will be on deck, even young children, unless prior notice is given.

- Table manners (including such niceties as pulling out chairs for the ladies and waiting until everyone is seated and grace has been said to start eating) can and should be encouraged.

- Televisions should be turned off and phones unanswered, taken off the hook, or (in the case of cell phones) turned off. This is a time to talk to one another, unhindered by a yammering TV or the intrusion of whoever decides to dial your number.

- Speaking of talking, the family table should be a place of warmth, respect, safety, genuine interest in what everyone has to say, and mutual support. If mealtimes are a hotbed of bickering and animosity, no one is going to want to show up. If the kids are having a little trouble with this, some role modeling of respectful conversation from Mom and Dad will speak volumes. And, if no one seems to have much to say, ask a few open-ended questions such as, "What was the high (or low) point of your day?"

- Finally, mealtimes can provide opportunities to talk with your children about the foods they (and you) eat and why some are definitely better than others. Obviously, teaching by example at the table—serving the foods you're discussing—also speaks volumes and helps set patterns that will continue long after children have left home to live on their own.

Endnotes

[1] Sally Squires, "Sweet But Not So Innocent? High-Fructose Corn Syrup, Ubiquitous in the American Diet, May Act More Like Fat Than Sugar in the Body," *Washington Post,* March 11, 2003.

[2] Center for Science in the Public Interest, "Sugar Intake Hit All-Time High in 1999," news release, May 18, 2000. See http://www.cspinet.org/new/sugar_limit.html.

[3] Findings from the ongoing Nurses' Health Study and the Health Professionals Follow-up Study, summarized in Walter Willett, *Eat, Drink and Be Healthy: The Harvard Medical School Guide to Healthy Eating* (New York: Fireside, 2001).

[4] C. S. Fuchs et al., "Dietary Fiber and the Risk of Colorectal Cancer and Adenoma in Women," *New England Journal of Medicine* 340 (1999): 169–176.

[5] Institute of Medicine, *Dietary Reference Intakes for Energy, Carbohydrate, Fiber, Fat, Fatty Acids, Cholesterol, Protein, and Amino Acids (Macronutrients).* See http://www.iom.edu/report.asp?id=4340.

[6] American Cancer Society, "Common Questions about Diet and Cancer." See http://www.cancer.org/docroot/ped/content/ped_3_2x_common_questions_about_diet_and_cancer.asp. (last accessed October 8, 2005).

[7] Harvard School of Public Health, "Fruits and Vegetables May Reduce Risk of Stroke: Findings Support Recommended 5 Servings a Day," news release, October 5, 1999. See http://www.hsph.harvard.edu/press/releases/press10051999.html.

[8] Harvard School of Public Health, "Fruits & Vegetables." See http://www.hsph.harvard.edu/nutritionsource/fruits.html (last accessed October 8, 2005).

Index

Antioxidants, 57–58

Atkins diet, 14

Calcium, 10, 56, 64

Calories
  empty, 5–6
  fat and, 46–48
  recommended daily amounts of,
    69–70
  storage of excess, 35–36
  sugar and, 5–6

Cancer
  effects of fruit and vegetables
    on, 30
  effects of whole grains on, 19

Carbohydrates, 1–2, 13–18, 21

Cardiovascular disease
  effects of fruit and vegetables
    on, 30
  effects of whole grains on, 19

Cataract
  effects of fruit and vegetables
    on, 30–31

Cholesterol, 23, 37–39, 49–51,
  70–71, 73
  high-density lipoproteins
    (HDL), 38–39, 42
  low-density lipoproteins
    (LDL), 38–39, 42

Coronary artery disease
  effects of omega-3 fatty acids
    on, 45

Diabetes
  effects of whole grains on, 19
  type 2; 22

Diet
  fruits and vegetables, 27–29, 32–34

Dietary fiber, 17, 21–26, 71, 73
  sources of, 24

Dietary supplements, 58–65
  and daily values, 62
  selecting, 60–65

Fast food, 49, 59, 86

Fat, 35–52
  "good," 43–45, 51–52
  role in the body, 35–36

Fatty acids, 37, 39–45

Fiber. See Dietary fiber

Folic acid, 19, 60, 64

Food Guide Pyramid, 14, 74–77

Fructose, 2

Fruit. See Diet, fruits and
  vegetables

Glucose, 1–2, 15–16

Glycemic index, 15–18

Glycemic load, 17–18

Heart disease. See Cardiovascular
  disease

Hyperactivity. See Sugar,
  hyperactivity and

Iron, 19, 60, 63, 64

Linoleic acid, 43

Linolenic acid, 43

Macular degeneration
    effects of fruit and vegetables
        on, 31
Minerals, 56. *See also* Dietary
    supplements
Monounsaturated fatty acids
    (MUFAs), 40, 41, 70–71
Nutrition Facts label, 8, 9, 25, 46–47,
    68–72
Omega-3 fatty acids, 43–45, 51
Omega-6 fatty acids, 43–44, 51
Partially hydrogenated, 41
Polyunsaturated fats
    (PUFAs), 40–42, 70–71
Portion size, 29, 80–82, 86–87
Protein, 31, 51, 71
Protein Power, 14
Restaurants, 85–87. *See also* Fast food
Saturated fats (SFAs), 39–40, 50, 71–
    71, 73
Starches, 13–16
Stroke
    effects of fruit and vegetables
        on, 30

Sucrose, 1–2
Sugar, 1–11
    effects on teeth of, 6–7
    hyperactivity and, 7
    invert, 3
    limiting intake of, 7, 71
    obesity and, 4–5
    types of, 1–3
Sugar Busters!, 14
Trans fatty acids, 42, 48–49
United States Pharmacopeia, 61
Vegetables. *See* Diet, fruits and
    vegetables
Vitamin C, 31, 55, 57, 60, 61,
    63–64
Vitamin E, 19, 31, 55, 57, 61,
    63–64
Vitamins, 54–55. *See also* Dietary
    supplements
Whole grains, 17
    benefits of, 18–19
    sources of, 19–20

GET THE *COMPLETE GUIDE TO FAMILY HEALTH, NUTRITION & FITNESS!*

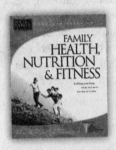

This comprehensive guide will help you take an active role in improving your health and well-being, as well as that of your entire family. It offers authoritative and current medical information in a convenient, easy-to-understand format. Taking a balanced, commonsense approach to the issue of health and wellness, this indispensable guide delivers helpful resources with an encouraging perspective.

OTHER FAITH AND FAMILY STRENGTHENERS FROM FOCUS ON THE FAMILY®

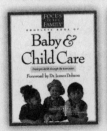

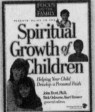

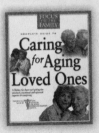

$6 REBATE

....

For a limited time you can get a $6.00 rebate on your purchase of *Complete Guide to Family Health, Nutrition, and Fitness*. Book must have been purchased in a retail store to qualify. Just return the completed rebate form, the original dated store receipt, and a photocopy of the UPC bar code from the book to: Complete Guide Rebate, Attn. Customer Service, 351 Executive Dr., Carol Stream, IL 60188.

Name: _____

Address: _____

_____

City:_____State:_____Zip:_____

Store where purchased: _____

E-mail address: _____

Signature: _____